Managing the Diabetic Foot

second edition

Michael E Edmonds MD, FRCP
Consultant Physician
Diabetic Foot Clinic
King's Diabetes Centre
King's College Hospital
London, UK

Alethea VM Foster
BA(Hons), PGCE, MChS, SRCh, Dip.Pod.M
Honorary Consultant Podiatrist
Diabetic Foot Clinic
King's Diabetes Centre
King's College Hospital
London, UK

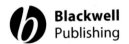

Blackwell
Publishing

First published 2000
Second edition 2005
3   2006

Library of Congress Cataloging-in-Publication Data
Edmonds, M. E.
   Managing the diabetic foot / Michael E. Edmonds, Alethea V.M.Foster.–2nd ed.
      p. ; cm.
   Includes bibliographical references and index.
   ISBN-13: 978-1-4051-2970-1 (alk. paper)
   ISBN-10: 1-4051-2970-0 (alk. paper)
   1. Foot–Ulcers. 2. Diabetes–Complications.
[DNLM: 1. Diabetic Foot–therapy. WK 835 E24m 2005] I. Foster, Alethea V. M. II. Title.
   RD563.E328 2005
   616.4'60–dc22

ISBN-13: 978-1-4051-2970-1
ISBN-10: 1-4051-2970-0

A catalogue record for this title is available from the British Library

Set in Unica
Design and layout by The Designers Collective Ltd. London
Printed and bound by Replika Press Pvt. Ltd, India
Commissioning Editor: Alison Brown
Development Editor: Rebecca Huxley
Production Controller: Kate Charman

For further information on Blackwell Publishing, visit our website:
http://www.blackwellpublishing.com

The publisher's policy is to use permanent paper from mills that operate a sustainable forestry policy, and which has been manufactured from pulp processed using acid-free and elementary chlorine-free practices. Furthermore, the publisher ensures that the text paper and cover board used have met acceptable environmental accreditation standards.

Contents

Acknowledgements

We are grateful to colleagues past and present, who include Simon Fraser, Huw Walters, Mary Blundell, Cathy Eaton, Mark Greenhill, Susie Spencer, Maureen McColgan-Bates, Mel Doxford, Sally Wilson, Adora Hatrapal, E Maelor Thomas, Mick Morris, John Philpott-Howard, Jim Wade, Andrew Hay, Robert Lewis, Anne-Marie Ryan, Irina Mantey, Robert Hills, Rachel Ben-Salem, Muriel Buxton-Thomas, Mazin Al-Janabi, Dawn Hurley, Stephanie Amiel, Stephen Thomas, Daniela Pitei, Anthony duVivier, Paul Baskerville, Anthony Giddings, Irving Benjamin, Mark Myerson, Paul Sidhu, Joydeep Sinha, Patricia Wallace, Gillian Cavell, Lesley Boys, Magdi Hanna, Sue Peat, Colin Roberts, David Goss, Colin Deane, Sue Snowdon, Ana Grenfell, Tim Cundy, Pat Ascott, Lindis Richards, Kate Spicer, Debbie Broome, Liz Hampton, Timothy Jemmott, Michelle Buckley, Rosalind Phelan, Audrey Edmonds, Maggie Boase, Maria Back, Avril Witherington, Daniel Rajan, Hisham Rashid, Karen Fairbairn, Ian Eltringham, Nina Petrova, Lindy Begg, Barbara Wall, Mark O'Brien, Stephen Edmonds, Sacha Andrews, Barry Pike, Charlotte Biggs, Robin Luff, Jane Preece, Briony Sloper, Christian Pankhurst, Jim Beaumont, Matthew McShane, Cheryl Clark, Marcelo Perez, Nicholas Cooley, Paul Baines, Patricia Yerbury, Anna Korzon Burakowska, David Ross, Jason Wilkins, David Evans, Carol Gayle, David Hopkins and two great stalwarts of the foot clinic, Peter Watkins and the late David Pyke. The Podiatry Managers and Community Podiatrists from Lambeth, Southwark and Lewisham have also contributed greatly to the work of the Foot Clinic at King's over many years. We are also grateful to Lee Sanders who was our co-author in writing A Practical Manual of Diabetic Foot Care.

We give special thanks to Yvonne Bartlett, Alex Dionysiou, David Langdon and Lucy Wallace from the Department of Medical Photography at King's and the late lamented Chelsea School of Chiropody and Barbara Wall for illustrations.

Lastly, we are grateful to our long-suffering editors, Rebecca Huxley and Alison Brown at Blackwell Science and Pete Wilder of The Designers Collective for their patience and understanding.

Preface to second edition

We shall not cease from exploration
And the end of all our exploring
Will be to arrive where we started
And know the place for the first time.

T.S. Eliot – *"Little Gidding"* (the last of his *Four Quartets*)

We have written the second edition to support and encourage all those people who valiantly care for patients with the diabetic foot – one of the most fascinating but challenging of all diabetic complications. Diabetic feet quickly reach the point of no return and it is extremely important to diagnose problems early and carry out rapid interventions. This is the only way to manage diabetic feet and to save them from amputation and it is a key theme of our second edition.

Since we wrote the first edition in 1999, there have been major changes in the way we look after diabetic feet and we highlight these advances in our second edition. In keeping with other diabetic foot clinics, we have noted a marked increase in the number of patients presenting with neuroischaemic feet. These are 'unforgiving' feet and management needs to be precise and prompt. We describe the increasingly intense and holistic multi-disciplinary care of these patients in 'fast-track' clinics. There is growing emphasis on the prevention of vascular events with the widespread prescription of statins, angiotensin-converting enzyme inhibitors and platelet antagonists. There have been advances in angioplasty, with many distal angioplasties now being carried out as day cases. There has also been progress in the care of the wound including free tissue transfer; and the VAC pump has been established as an important treatment for large ulcers and postoperative wounds. Advances have been made in Charcot osteoarthropathy both in surgical internal stabilisation as well as in the development of external means of stabilisation such as the Charcot Restraint Orthotic Walker. Progress has been achieved in the management of painful peripheral neuropathy.

We continue to describe simple investigations and techniques of which we have had experience and which are readily available in any hospital or clinic that looks after diabetic patients with foot problems. We refer to patients throughout the book as "he" simply because more men than women seem to develop diabetic foot ulcers.

We have not endeavoured to produce a complete description of every aspect of the diabetic foot and we have deliberately not cited references but given a further reading list. We have also added an appendix of differential diagnosis lists for common presentations and hope this will be useful. Finally, we hope that this book will aid practitioners in their implementation of published guidelines which advise on the care of diabetic feet including the NICE (National Institute of Clinical Excellence) guidelines and the National Service Framework for Diabetes.

We must now accept that diabetes is pandemic and this will inevitably lead to an increase in the number of diabetic foot problems. However, amputations can be avoided by early diagnosis and prompt management and we hope that this book will improve survival of the diabetic foot in the 21st century.

Mike Edmonds
Ali Foster
London, February 2005

Chapter 1

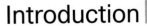

Introduction

NEW APPROACH TO THE DIABETIC FOOT

Three great pathologies come together in the diabetic foot: neuropathy, ischaemia and infection. Their combined impact is so great that it causes more amputations than any other lower limb disease. Although there have been many advances in the management of the diabetic foot, it nevertheless remains a major global public health problem. All over the world health-care systems have failed the diabetic foot patient; however, amputations are not inevitable. As diabetic foot problems quickly reach the point of no return, it is vital to diagnose them early and provide rapid and intensive treatment. Furthermore, it is important to achieve early recognition of the at-risk foot so as to institute prompt preventive measures. The multidisciplinary foot clinic can reduce the numbers of amputations and has been developed as a successful model of care throughout the world.

The aim of this book is to enable practitioners to take a new approach to the diabetic foot by early diagnosis and treatment. It attempts to give enough simple practical information to enable them to understand the natural history of the diabetic foot and to improve outcomes. This fundamental approach is built on a simple staging system based upon the natural history of the diabetic foot and developed to provide a framework for early diagnosis and management. Other staging systems are in use and may have their merits. The simple staging system covers the whole spectrum of diabetic foot disease but nevertheless emphasises the development of the foot ulcer as a pivotal event demanding urgent and aggressive management. Staging, however, does not imply automatic progression to the next stage.

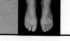

Assessment of the foot
Neuropathy
Ischaemia
Deformity
Callus
Swelling
Skin breakdown
Infection
Necrosis

Table 1.1
Eight clinical features in the assessment of the foot.

There are four main themes running throughout the book.
- Easy, practical assessment of the foot, looking for eight clinical features (Table 1.1)
- Simple classification of the diabetic foot, into the neuropathic and neuroischaemic foot
- Simple staging system, describing six specific stages in the natural history of the diabetic foot (Table 1.2)
- Simple management plan for each stage, outlining six aspects of early intervention and patient treatment, within a multidisciplinary framework (Table 1.3).

Thus, the overall approach to the diabetic foot starts with a simple assessment to enable the practitioner to make a basic classification and staging. This book describes full details of practical management for each stage in the appropriate chapter with one colour-coded chapter for each of the six stages. A short appendix describes the differential diagnosis of common presentations.

The book contains sufficient, easily accessible information to enable the practitioner to make rapid, effective decisions which will prevent deterioration and progression to amputation.

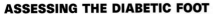

ASSESSING THE DIABETIC FOOT

The staging system is based on a simple assessment of the foot, which should take no longer than 5 minutes. There is a specific search for eight factors as shown in Table 1.1. Many of these features can be detected by an examination which includes:

- Simple inspection
- Palpation
- Sensory testing.

A complicated examination is not necessary. This chapter describes the search for these individual features and then presents an integrated examination. It is often helpful to detect abnormalities by comparing one foot with the other.

Shoe inspection should be included in the foot assessment and is described in Chapter 2.

Neuropathy

Neuropathy is the most common complication of diabetes affecting 50% of all diabetic patients. Although it may present with tingling and a feeling of numbness, it is asymptomatic in the majority of patients and neuropathy will only be detected by clinical examination. An important indication of neuropathy will be a patient who fails to complain of pain, even when significant foot lesions are present. Painless ulceration is definite evidence of a peripheral neuropathy.

The presentation of peripheral neuropathy is related to dysfunction of sensory, motor and autonomic nerves. Simple inspection will usually reveal signs of motor and autonomic neuropathy but sensory neuropathy must be detected by screening or by a simple sensory examination.

Motor neuropathy

The classical sign of a motor neuropathy is a high medial longitudinal arch, leading to prominent metatarsal heads and pressure points over the plantar forefoot (Fig. 1.1). In severe cases, pressure points also develop over the apices and dorsal interphalangeal joints of associated claw toes. However, claw toe is a

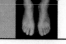
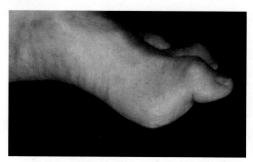

Fig. 1.1
Neuropathic foot showing motor neuropathy with high medial longitudinal arch, leading to prominent metatarsal heads and pressure points over the plantar forefoot.

common deformity and may not always be related to a motor neuropathy. It may be caused by wearing unsuitable shoes or trauma or may be congenital.

Complicated assessment of motor power in the foot or leg is not usually necessary, but it is advisable to test dorsiflexion of the foot to detect a foot drop secondary to a common peroneal nerve palsy. This is usually unilateral and will affect the patient's gait.

Autonomic neuropathy

The classical signs of autonomic neuropathy are:

- Dry skin with fissuring (Fig. 1.2)
- Distended veins over the dorsum of the foot and ankle (Fig. 1.3).

The dry skin is secondary to decreased sweating. The sweating loss normally occurs in a stocking distribution, which can extend up to the knee. The distended veins are secondary to arteriovenous shunting associated with autonomic neuropathy.

Sensory neuropathy

Sensory neuropathy can be simply detected by:

- Monofilaments (Fig. 1.4) or
- Neurothesiometry (Fig. 1.5).

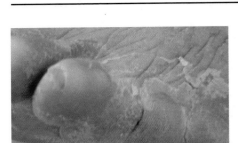

Fig. 1.2
Dry skin with fissures.

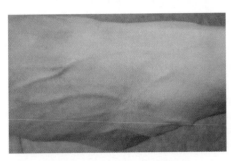

Fig. 1.3
Distended veins over the dorsum of the foot and ankle.

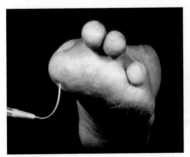

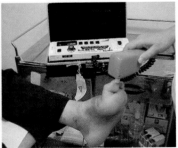

Fig. 1.4
Nylon monofilament buckles at a force of 10 g when applied perpendicularly to the foot. If the patient cannot feel this pressure then protective sensation has been lost.

Fig. 1.5
Neurothesiometer, a device which when applied to the foot delivers a vibratory stimulus which increases as the voltage is raised.

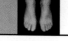

If these are not available, then a simple clinical examination detecting sensation to light touch using a cotton wisp and vibration using a 128-Hz tuning fork will suffice, comparing a proximal site with a distal site to confirm a symmetrical stocking-like distribution of the neuropathy.

The advantage of the assessment with monofilaments or neurothesiometry is that it detects patients who have lost protective pain sensation and are therefore susceptible to foot ulceration.

A simple technique for detecting neuropathy is to use a nylon monofilament, which, when applied perpendicular to the foot, buckles at a given force of 10 grams. The filament should be pressed against several sites including the plantar aspects of the first toe, the first, third and fifth metatarsal heads, the plantar surface of the heel and the dorsum of the foot. The filament should not be applied at any site until callus has been removed. If the patient cannot feel the filament at a tested area, then significant neuropathy is present and protective pain sensation is lost. After using a monofilament on ten consecutive patients, there should be a recovery time of 24 hours before further usage.

The degree of neuropathy can be further quantified by the use of the neurothesiometer. When applied to the foot, this device delivers a vibratory stimulus, which increases as the voltage is raised. The vibration threshold increases with age, but, for practical purposes, any patient unable to feel a vibratory stimulus of 25 volts is at risk of ulceration.

A small number of patients have a small-fibre neuropathy with impaired pain and temperature perception but with intact touch and vibration. They are prone to ulceration and thermal traumas but test normally with filaments and neurothesiometer, and a clinical assessment of light touch and vibration is normal. As yet, there is no inexpensive method of detecting and quantifying small-fibre neuropathy. However, a simple assessment of cold sensation can be made by placing a cold tuning fork on the patient's foot and leg.

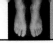

Ischaemia

Ischaemia results from atherosclerosis of the arteries of the leg. Claudication is often absent because of concomitant neuropathy. Ulceration or necrosis is the commonest presentation of ischaemia. The skin is thin, shiny and without hair. There is atrophy of the subcutaneous tissue.

In critical ischaemia, skin colour is often a dusky red or cyanotic blue because impaired perfusion has resulted in stagnation of blood in dilated arterioles. In acute ischaemia, the foot is pale, often with purplish mottling, and the nail beds are white or blueish.

The most important manoeuvre to detect ischaemia is the palpation of foot pulses, an examination which is often undervalued.

- The dorsalis pedis pulse is lateral to the extensor hallucis longus tendon on the dorsum of the foot (Fig. 1.6a)
- The posterior tibial pulse is below and behind the medial malleolus (Fig. 1.6b)
- If either of these foot pulses can be felt then it is highly unlikely that there is significant ischaemia.

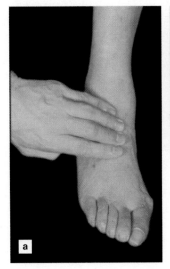

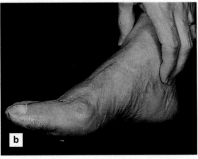

Fig. 1.6
(a) Palpation of dorsalis pedis pulse on the dorsum of the foot. (b) Palpation of the posterior tibial pulse.

A small hand-held Doppler can be used to confirm the presence of pulses and to quantify the vascular supply. Used together with a sphygmomanometer, the brachial systolic pressure and ankle systolic pressure can be measured, and the pressure index, which is the ratio of ankle systolic pressure to brachial systolic pressure, can be calculated. In normal subjects, the pressure index is usually > 1, but in the presence of ischaemia is < 1. Thus, absence of pulses and a pressure index of < 1 confirms ischaemia. Conversely, the presence of pulses and a pressure index of > 1 rules out ischaemia. This has important implications for management, namely that macrovascular disease is not an important factor and further vascular investigations are not necessary.

Many diabetic patients have medial arterial calcification, giving an artificially elevated systolic pressure, even in the presence of ischaemia. It is thus difficult to assess the diabetic foot when the pulses are not palpable, but the pressure index is > 1. There are two explanations:

- The examiner may have missed the pulses, particularly in an oedematous foot, and should go back to palpate the foot after the arteries have been located by Doppler ultrasound
- If the pulses remain impalpable, then ischaemia probably exists in the presence of medial wall calcification. It is then necessary to use other methods to assess flow in the arteries of the foot, such as examining the pattern of the Doppler arterial waveform or measuring transcutaneous oxygen tension or toe systolic pressures (see Chapter 4).

Despite the difficulties of interpreting ankle systolic pressures in the presence of medial calcification, a low pressure index of 0.5 or less indicates severe ischaemia whether the patient is calcified or not.

Deformity

It is important to recognize deformity in the diabetic foot. Deformity often leads to bony prominences, which are associated with high mechanical pressures on the overlying skin. This results in ulceration, particularly in the absence of protective pain sensation and when shoes are unsuitable. Ideally, the deformity should be recognized early and accommodated in properly fitting shoes before ulceration occurs.

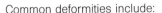

Common deformities include:
- Claw toes
- Pes cavus
- Hallux rigidus
- Hallux valgus
- Hammer toe
- Mallet toe
- Fibro-fatty padding depletion
- Charcot foot
- Deformities related to previous trauma and surgery
- Nail deformities.

Claw toes

Claw toes (Fig. 1.7) have fixed flexion deformities at the interphalangeal joints and are associated with callus and ulceration of the apices and dorsal aspects of the interphalangeal joints. Although claw toes may be related to neuropathy, they are often unrelated, especially when the clawing is unilateral and associated with trauma or surgery of the forefoot. Claw toes may result from acute rupture of the plantar fascia.

Pes Cavus

Normally the dorsum of the foot is domed due to the medial longitudinal arch which extends between the first metatarsal head and the calcaneus. When it is abnormally high, the deformity is called pes cavus and the abnormal distribution of pressure leads to excessive callus formation under the metatarsal heads (Fig. 1.1).

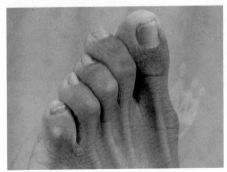

Fig. 1.7
Claw toes.

9

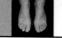
Hallux rigidus

This leads to limited joint mobility of the first metatarso-phalangeal joint with loss of dorsiflexion and results in excessive forces on the plantar surface of the first toe, causing callus formation.

Hallux valgus

Hallux valgus is a deformity of the first metatarso-phalangeal joint with lateral deviation of the hallux and a medial prominence on the margin of the foot. This site is particularly vulnerable in the neuroischaemic foot and frequently breaks down under pressure from a tight shoe (Fig. 1.8).

Hammer toe

Hammer toe is a flexion deformity of the proximal interphalangeal joint of a lesser toe with hyperextension of the distal interphalangeal joint (Fig. 1.9). The toe is at risk of dorsal ulceration.

Mallet toe

This deformity is a flexion contracture at the distal interphalangeal joint.

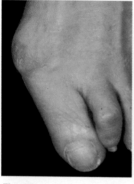

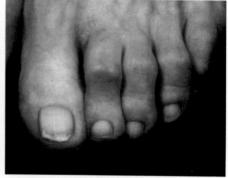

Fig. 1.8
Hallux valgus with erythema at first metatarso-phalangeal joint from tight shoe.

Fig. 1.9
Hammer toes (2nd, 3rd and 4th toes) with hyperflexion of the proximal interphalangeal joints and hyperextension of the distal interphalangeal joints.

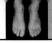

Fibro-fatty padding depletion

The plantar soft-tissue overlying the metatarsal heads is frequently pushed forward or destroyed by previous ulceration or infection. This leads to depletion of padding and raised plantar pressures.

Charcot foot

Bone and joint damage in the metatarso-tarsal region is the commonest site of involvement and leads to two classical deformities:

- Rocker-bottom deformity (Fig. 1.10) in which there is displacement and subluxation of the tarsus downwards
- Medial convexity, which results from displacement of the talonavicular joint or from tarso-metatarsal dislocation.

Both are often associated with a bony prominence which is very prone to ulceration. Healing is notoriously difficult. If these deformities are not diagnosed early and accommodated in properly fitting footwear, ulceration at vulnerable pressure points often develops (Fig. 1.11). The Charcot foot is fully discussed in Chapter 8.

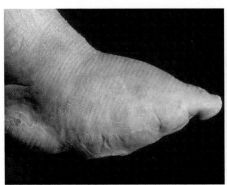

Fig. 1.10
Charcot foot showing rocker-bottom deformity.

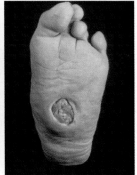

Fig. 1.11
Ulceration over bony prominence on the plantar surface of a rocker-bottom deformity.

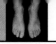

Deformities related to previous trauma and surgery

Deformities of the hip and fractures of the tibia or fibula lead to leg-shortening and hence abnormal gait, which predisposes to foot ulceration.

Ray amputations remove the toe together with part of the metatarsal. They are usually very successful but disturb the biomechanics of the foot leading to high pressure under the adjacent metatarsal heads. Removal of the 5th ray may lead to varus deformity of the foot if the 5th metatarsal base and its muscle attachments are not preserved. After amputation of a toe, deformities are often seen in adjoining toes (Fig. 1.12).

Nail deformities

It is important to inspect the nails closely as these may become the site of ulceration. Thickened nails are common in the population at large and may lead to ulceration.

Ingrowing toe nail (onychocryptosis) arises when the nail plate is excessively wide and thin, or develops a convex deformity, putting pressure on the tissues at the nail edge. Callus builds up in response to pressure and inflammation. Eventually, usually after incorrect nail cutting or trauma, the nail penetrates the flesh (see page 29, Figs. 2.6 and 2.7).

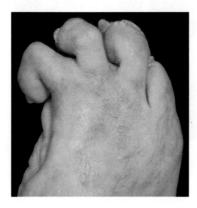

Fig. 1.12
Deformity of toe adjacent to amputated first toe.

Callus

This is a thickened area of epidermis which develops at sites of pressure, shear and friction. It should not be allowed to become excessive as callus is a common forerunner of ulceration in the presence of neuropathy.

Swelling

Swelling of the tissues of the foot is a major factor predisposing to ulceration, and often exacerbates a tight fit inside poorly fitting shoes. It also impedes healing of established ulcers.

Swelling may be bilateral or unilateral.

Bilateral swelling

This is usually secondary to:

- Cardiac failure
- Renal impairment
- Venous insufficiency (sometimes unilateral)
- Diabetic neuropathy when it is related to increased arterial blood flow and arteriovenous shunting and is referred to as neuropathic oedema.

Unilateral swelling

This is usually associated with local pathology in the foot or leg. Causes are:

- Infection, when it is usually associated with erythema and a break in the skin (Figs. 1.13a and b)
- Charcot foot (a unilateral hot, red, swollen foot is often the first sign) (Fig. 1.14) – the swelling can extend to the knee
- Gout, which may also present as a hot, red, swollen foot
- Trauma, sprain or fracture
- Deep vein thrombosis, venous insufficiency or lymphoedema secondary to malignancy
- Localized collection of blood or pus which may present as a fluctuant swelling.

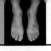

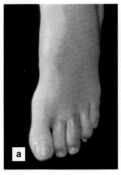
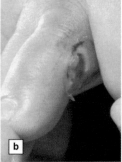
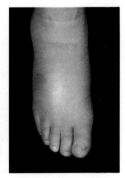

Fig. 1.13
(a) Erythema and swelling of the third toe spreading up the foot. (b) Interdigital ulcer as source of sepsis with cellulitis and blue discolouration adjacent to ulcer.

Fig. 1.14
Acute stage of Charcot foot; erythema and swelling of the dorsum of the foot.

Skin breakdown

An active search should be made for breaks in the skin over the entire surface of the foot and ankle, not forgetting the areas between the toes and at the back of the heel. Toes should be gently held apart for inspection (Fig. 1.13b). If jerked apart, this can split the skin. The classical sign of tissue breakdown is the foot ulcer. However, fissures (Fig. 1.15) and bullae/blisters (Fig. 1.16) also represent breakdown of the skin.

Some lesions will be obvious; others will make their presence known by their complications such as:
- Discharge or exudate
- Colour changes under callus or nail plate
- Pain or discomfort
- Swelling
- Warmth
- Erythema.

Infection

When skin breakdown develops, it may act as a portal of entry for infection (see Chapter 5). A close inspection for signs of infection should be made. These include purulent discharge from the lesion and erythema, swelling and warmth of the toe or foot (Fig. 1.17).

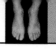

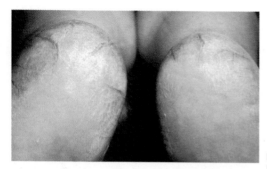

Fig. 1.15
Fissures of heel.

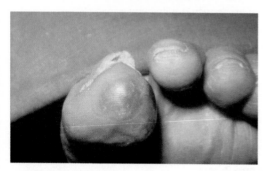

Fig. 1.16
Bulla over apex of first toe.

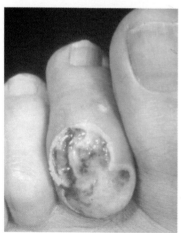

Fig. 1.17
Ulceration, cellulitis and purulent discharge from toe.

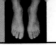
Necrosis

Finally, lesions of skin breakdown may progress to underlying necrosis (Fig. 1.18). This can be identified by the presence of black or brown devitalized tissue (see Chapter 6).

Integrated examination

In practice, the examination of the foot should be divided into three main parts: inspection, palpation and neurological assessment.

Inspection

The foot should be fully inspected including dorsum, sole, back of the heel and interdigital areas with a full assessment of:

- Colour (as an indicator of ischaemia)
- Deformity
- Swelling
- Callus
- Skin breakdown
- Infection
- Necrosis.

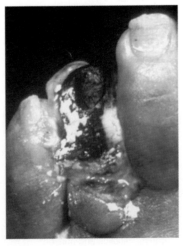

Fig. 1.18
Wet necrosis of toe (see also Chapter 6).

Palpation

Pulses should be palpated and skin temperature compared between both feet with the back of the examining hand. The measurement of skin temperature is particularly helpful in the management of the Charcot foot, when a digital skin thermometer is useful (see Chapter 8).

Neurological assessment

Peripheral neuropathy should be detected either by using the monofilament or neurothesiometer or by performing a simple sensory examination as described above.

After completing this basic examination, it will now be possible to classify the diabetic foot and to make the appropriate staging in its natural history.

CLASSIFYING THE DIABETIC FOOT

For practical purposes, the diabetic foot can be divided into two entities, the neuropathic foot and the ischaemic foot. However, ischaemia is nearly always associated with neuropathy, and the ischaemic foot is best called the neuroischaemic foot. The purely ischaemic foot, with no concomitant neuropathy, is rarely seen in diabetic patients and its management is the same as for the neuroischaemic foot except when sharp debriding which may be painful in the absence of neuropathy.

It is essential to differentiate between the neuropathic and the neuroischaemic foot as their management will differ.

Infection is the most frequent complication of ulceration in both the neuropathic and neuroischaemic foot. It is important to diagnose it early and intervene rapidly. It is responsible for considerable tissue necrosis in the diabetic foot and this is the main reason for major amputation.

The neuropathic foot

- It is a warm, well perfused foot with bounding pulses due to arteriovenous shunting and distended dorsal veins
- Sweating is diminished, the skin may be dry and prone to fissuring, and any callus present tends to be hard and dry

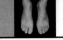

- Toes may be clawed and the foot arch raised
- Ulceration commonly develops on the sole of the foot, associated with neglected callus and high plantar pressures
- Despite the good circulation, necrosis can develop secondary to severe infection
- It is also prone to bone and joint problems (the Charcot foot)
- As patients are followed for many years in the diabetic foot clinic, the neuropathic foot often develops ischaemia and becomes a neuroischaemic foot.

The Neuroischaemic foot

- It is a cool, pulseless foot with reduced perfusion and almost invariably has neuropathy
- The colour of the severely ischaemic foot can be a deceptively healthy pink or red, caused by dilatation of capillaries in an attempt to improve perfusion. If severely infected, the ischaemic foot may feel deceptively warm
- It may also be complicated by swelling, often secondary to cardiac failure or renal failure
- The most frequent presentation is that of ulceration. Ischaemic ulcers are commonly seen on the margins of the foot, including the tips of the toes and the areas around the back of the heel, and are usually caused by trauma or by wearing unsuitable shoes, which do not accommodate deformity
- Intermittent claudication and rest pain may be absent because of neuropathy and the distal distribution of the arterial disease to the leg
- Even if neuropathy is present and plantar pressures are high, plantar ulceration is rare, probably because the foot does not develop heavy callus, which requires good blood flow
- It develops necrosis in the presence of infection or if tissue perfusion is critically diminished.

Throughout the world, type 2 diabetes is becoming more highly prevalent, leading to complications of peripheral vascular disease and neuropathy. This leads to the neuroischaemic foot, which has now become the most frequently encountered type of foot to present in the

United Kingdom. There has been a change of predominance from neuropathic to neuroischaemic feet as people present more readily with ischaemic disease and live longer with feet which may be salvaged by bypass or angioplasty but are still challenging to manage.

THE NATURAL HISTORY OF THE DIABETIC FOOT

The natural history of the diabetic foot can be divided into six stages as shown in Table 1.2.

Stage 1

The foot is not at risk. The patient does not have the risk factors of neuropathy, ischaemia, deformity, callus and swelling rendering him vulnerable to foot ulcers.

Stage 2

The patient has developed one or more of the risk factors for ulceration of the foot, which may be divided into the neuropathic foot (Fig. 1.19) and the neuroischaemic foot (Fig. 1.20).

Stage 3

The foot has a skin breakdown. This is usually an ulcer, but because some minor injuries such as blisters, splits or grazes have a propensity to become ulcers, they are included in Stage 3. Ulceration is usually on the plantar surface in the neuropathic foot (Fig. 1.21) and usually on the margin in the neuroischaemic foot (Fig. 1.22).

Staging the diabetic foot	
Stage	Clinical condition
1	Normal
2	High-risk
3	Ulcerated
	Infected
5	Necrotic
6	Unsalvageable

Table 1.2
Staging the diabetic foot.

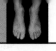
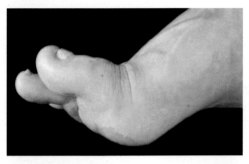

Fig. 1.19
Neuropathic foot showing motor neuropathy with high medial longitudinal arch, leading to prominent metatarsal heads and pressure points over the plantar forefoot.

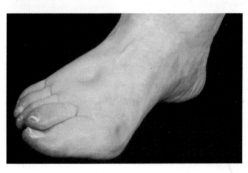

Fig. 1.20
Neuroischaemic foot with pitting oedema secondary to cardiac failure. There is also hallux valgus and erythema from pressure of tight shoe on the medial aspect of the first metatarso-phalangeal joint

Stage 4
The ulcer has developed infection with the presence of cellulitis which can complicate both the neuropathic (Fig. 1.23) and the neuroischaemic foot (Fig. 1.24).

Stage 5
Necrosis has supervened. In the neuropathic foot, infection is usually the cause (Fig. 1.25); in the neuroischaemic foot, infection is still the most common reason for tissue destruction (Fig. 1.26) although ischaemia contributes.

Stage 6
The foot cannot be saved and will need a major amputation.

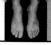

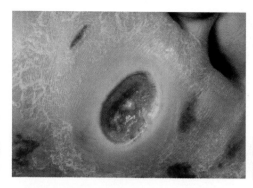

Fig. 1.21
Neuropathic foot with
plantar ulcer surrounded
by callus.

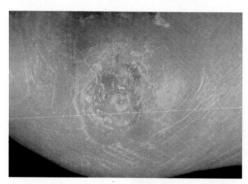

Fig. 1.22
Ulcer over medial aspect
of 1st metatarso-
phalangeal joint of a
neuroischaemic foot.

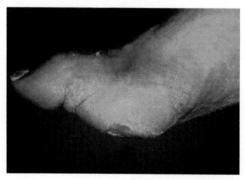

Fig. 1.23
Cellulitis complicating
neuropathic plantar ulcer.

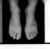

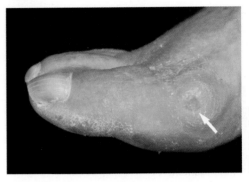

Fig. 1.24
Cellulitis in a neuroischaemic foot with ulcer (arrowed) that is the portal of entry for infection.

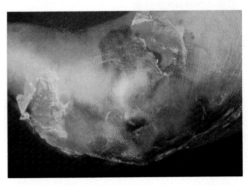

Fig. 1.25
Necrosis indicated by blue–black discolouration surrounded by cellulitis and haemorrhage in a neuropathic foot.

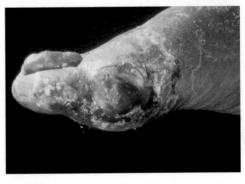

Fig. 1.26
Ulceration, discharge and necrosis in a neuroischaemic foot.

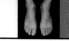

Most diabetic foot problems will fall under one of the six stages. Three exceptions to this rule are the Charcot foot, neuropathic fracture and painful neuropathy (see Chapter 8).

MULTIDISCIPLINARY MANAGEMENT

The aim in managing diabetic foot problems is always to keep the patient at as low a stage as possible. At each stage of the diabetic foot, it is necessary to intervene early and take control of the foot to prevent further progression. Management will be considered under the headings shown in Table 1.3. The subsequent chapters will fully describe each aspect of management for each stage.

The multidisciplinary diabetic foot team

A foot ulcer is a sign of systemic disease and successful management of the diabetic foot needs the expertise of a multidisciplinary team which provides integrated care focused in a diabetic foot clinic. No one person can take control of the diabetic foot. Members of the team will include physician, podiatrist, nurse, orthotist, radiologist and surgeon. It is helpful if the team works closely together, within the focus of the diabetic foot clinic, and also meets regularly for ward rounds and X-ray conferences. Each team member should be available quickly in an emergency. Some roles may overlap, depending on local expertise and interest. All members

Six aspects of patient treatment
Wound control
Microbiological control
Mechanical control
Vascular control
Metabolic control
Educational control

Table 1.3
Six aspects of patient treatment, within a multidisciplinary framework.

of the team must realise that neuropathy often delays the patient's presentation because he does not have pain and may not take the lesion seriously. This is a mistake that can also be made by his medical attendants, who have been educated in a diagnostic process that assumes pain is a reliable indicator of the seriousness of the presentation. This is not true in the diabetic foot.

Day to day multidisciplinary treatment is carried out by podiatrist, nurse, orthotist and physician in the diabetic foot clinic. Further multidisciplinary management can be achieved by holding regular joint clinics when appropriate groups of patients are assembled in the diabetic foot clinic. At King's, these are held regularly with vascular and orthopaedic surgeons. Through these specialist clinics, it is possible to organise a 'fast-track' service with a 'one-stop' visit. In the joint clinic with the vascular surgeon, the need for angiography and angioplasty can be rapidly agreed upon and promptly carried out as a day case where appropriate. The results can be quickly reviewed and further action taken.

The diabetic foot clinic should provide rapid access, early diagnosis and prompt help for patients with foot problems. Such patients will need close follow up for the rest of their lives. Emergency services can be run concurrently with routine clinics so that patients with new ulcers, pain or discolouration can be seen the same day (in accordance with the National Institute of Clinical Excellence (NICE) guidelines for managing the diabetic foot). Rapid admission to hospital for the foot in jeopardy can also be arranged through this emergency service. Emergency services should be available in office hours from Monday to Friday. Outside these hours, special arrangements should be made with the local casualty department to manage diabetic feet in trouble.

Chapter 2

Managing Stage 1: the normal foot

PRESENTATION AND DIAGNOSIS

The foot has none of the risk factors for foot ulcers, namely, neuropathy, ischaemia, deformity, callus and swelling, and the diagnosis of Stage 1 is made by excluding these risk factors.

Techniques for their assessment have been described in the Introduction, and they should be carried out when the patient presents for annual review.

MANAGEMENT

The aim of management is to keep the foot at Stage 1. The following components of multidisciplinary management are important:
- Mechanical control
- Metabolic control
- Educational control.

This stage does not have any skin breakdown or ischaemia: therefore, wound, microbiological and vascular control are not relevant.

Mechanical control

Mechanical control is based upon wearing the correct footwear. It also involves the diagnosis and treatment of common problems affecting the biomechanics of the foot.

Correct footwear

If shoes are the wrong size or style, they can permanently damage the feet, and lead to deformity callus and ulceration.

All people at Stage 1 will be wearing their own shoes. Therefore, advice about footwear purchase is necessary and patients should be told the principles of good footwear (Table 2.1) (Figs. 2.1, 2.2). If possible, shoes should be purchased on approval and checked by a health-care professional. Trainer styles (Fig. 2.3) are useful.

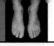
Good shoe guide

The toe box should be sufficiently long, broad and deep to accommodate the toes without pressing on them, with a clear space between the apices of the toes and the toe box so that the toes are not too cramped to function

Shoes should fasten with adjustable lace, strap or Velcro high on the foot. (When the lace is fastened, the foot is firmly held inside the shoe thus reducing the frictional forces when the patient walks and preventing the foot from sliding forwards and jamming the toes against the toe box.) Shoes should be foot shaped

The heel of the shoe should be under 5 cm high to avoid weight being thrown forward on to metatarsal heads (Figs. 2.2 and 2.3)

The inner lining of the shoe should be smooth

Shoes should be purchased in the afternoon because feet swell a little during the day

Stockings or socks should always be worn with shoes to avoid blisters. Socks with prominent seams should be worn inside out and socks with holes should be replaced

Table 2.1
Good shoe guide.

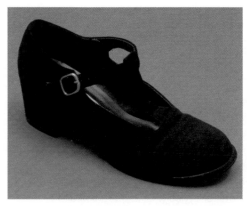

Fig. 2.1
A 'good' woman's shoe with low heel, generous toe box and restraining strap fastening high on the foot.

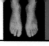

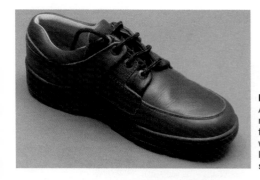

Fig. 2.2
A good 'high-street'
man's shoe. Lace holds
foot back during walking,
with roomy toe box and
low heel. The shoe is the
shape of the foot.

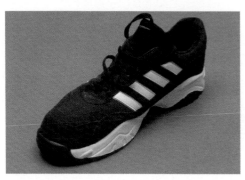

Fig. 2.3
'High-street' trainer-style
shoes.

Shoes should be part of the foot assessment and features of a
bad shoe are shown in Fig. 2.4.

Minor foot problems

In achieving mechanical control, it is important to diagnose common
foot problems which are not peculiar to diabetes but are very
common in the population at large. Most people in Stage 1 will be
able to cut their own nails (Table 2.2). However, specific nail and
other minor foot problems will need treatment. Minor foot problems
can become major problems in the future unless they are diagnosed
early and treated.

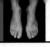

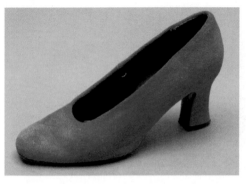

Fig. 2.4
A 'bad' woman's shoe. Heel is too high, toe box is cramped and it has no fastening.

Patients who can safely cut their own toe nails
Pain-free normal nails with no pathology
Can see feet clearly
Can reach feet
Have been taught correct nail cutting techniques

Table 2.2
Patients who can safely cut their own toe nails.

ONYCHOGRYPHOSIS This is thickening of the nail with deformity (Fig. 2.5). The cause is a previous insult to the nail bed and it is necessary to file down the nail regularly otherwise it may grow at an angle and penetrate adjoining tissue. Gryphotic nails should be treated by a podiatrist who will regularly reduce the bulk of the nail.

ONYCHOCRYPTOSIS This is ingrowing toenail, often due to poor toe nail cutting technique or trauma. A splinter of nail, left behind by incomplete cutting or attempts to remove the corners of the nail, penetrates the nail sulcus (the groove of flesh at the side of the nail plate).

The offending splinter of nail (Fig. 2.6) should be removed (Fig. 2.7) and the ragged edge of the nail filed smooth. Unless the splinter of nail is removed, the flesh will be penetrated and infection supervenes. The lesion will not heal and paronychia may develop.

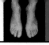

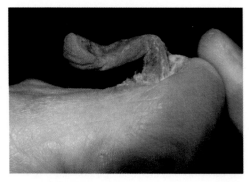

Fig. 2.5
Onychogryphosis.

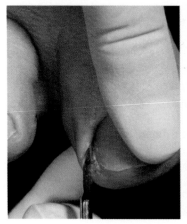

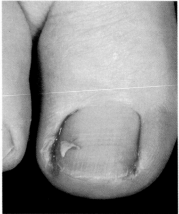

Fig. 2.6
Onychocryptosis. A spike of nail has been 'left behind' after cutting.

Fig. 2.7
Onychocryptosis. The offending spike has been removed and lies on the nail plate.

If the problem does not resolve, partial nail avulsion under local anaesthetic and phenolysation of the nail matrix may be necessary although it can take several weeks to heal. It is safe to carry this out in a Stage 1 diabetic patient who, by definition, has good peripheral circulation.

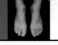

ONYCHOMYCOSIS Fungal infection can cause whitish or yellowish discolouration of the nail plate which frequently becomes thickened and crumbly (Fig. 2.8).

The majority of infections are caused by dermatophytes or yeasts. Eradication is difficult. Unless the condition is spreading, painful or cosmetically unacceptable, palliative care is best. The bulk of the nail should be reduced at regular intervals. Active treatment involves topical or systemic agents. Systemic agents may cause side-effects. Terbinafine is the drug of choice.

INVOLUTED TOE NAILS These have an excessive lateral curvature and trap epithelial cells which accumulate in the sulcus and become painful (Fig. 2.9). The sulcus should be gently cleared with a Black's file (a small file specially designed to fit into the sulcus). Removal of the edge of the nail is also helpful.

SUBUNGUAL HAEMATOMA This follows trauma to the nail. Blood collects under the nail plate causing a red, purple or black discolouration. This may be painful. A large collection of blood can loosen the entire nail plate.

The haematoma can be drained by making a small hole in the nail plate with a scalpel or with a podiatrist's nail drill. If the nail plate is loose, it is best to cut it back before it catches on the hose and causes further trauma.

TINEA PEDIS This can present in several ways: moist, cracked areas with whitish macerated skin between the toes, a dry, scaly hyperkeratotic area or a vesicular itchy rash (Fig. 2.10) are all presentations.

Canesten spray (clotrimazole 1% in 30% isopropyl alcohol) or cream may be prescribed, which should be continued for 2 weeks after resolution of symptoms to avoid relapse. For other parts of the foot, Canesten cream can be applied. Whitfield's ointment is useful. Tinactin (tolnaftate) and Mycil (chlorphenesin) can be bought over the counter in powder or cream formulations.

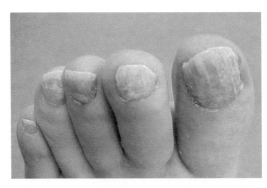

Fig. 2.8
Onychomychosis.

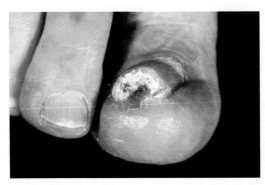

Fig. 2.9
Involuted first toe nail.

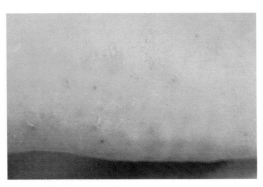

Fig. 2.10
Tinea pedis presenting
as an itchy vesicular
rash.

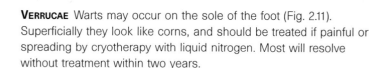

VERRUCAE Warts may occur on the sole of the foot (Fig. 2.11). Superficially they look like corns, and should be treated if painful or spreading by cryotherapy with liquid nitrogen. Most will resolve without treatment within two years.

CORNS These are areas where, in response to pressure or friction, the stratum corneum is thicker than in adjoining areas and has a deeper nucleus. Corns between the toes are soft and white.

Corns should be removed by a podiatrist and efforts made to reduce abnormal mechanical forces with good footwear.

BULLAE/BLISTERS Bullae are superficial fluid-filled sacs which develop when the skin is traumatized. The usual causes are inadequate footwear or failing to wear socks. If the feet and shoes and socks are wet, then blistering is more likely to develop.

If the bulla is small and flaccid, it can be cleaned and covered with a sterile dressing. If large and tense, it should be lanced with a scalpel to release the contents before dressing. Aspiration with a syringe is less useful, because the hole may seal and the bulla may become tense again.

CHILBLAINS These are localized inflammatory lesions, provoked by cold. They present as dusky red swellings in the acute stage and, in the chronic stage, as purple lesions on the toes. They are best prevented by making sure that the feet are well protected from the cold.

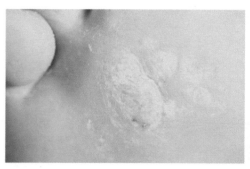

Fig. 2.11
Verucca pedis over the fourth metatarsal head.

TRAUMAS Superficial cuts and graz(..)
antiseptic and covered with a sterile (..)
should keep a first-aid box at home w(..)
dressings, tape and antiseptic cream to(..)

Any foot problem, no matter how app(..)
healing well within 48 hours should be trea(..)

DRY SKIN AND FISSURES It is essential for peop(..)
after the condition of the skin and to keep it cl(..)
scales, hyperkeratosis and cracks. This can be (..) (..)egular
washing, application of emollient to dry skin, and (..)(..)tic
debridement of hyperkeratosis. Clearing the edges of fissures to
achieve closure is important. Many ulcers can be prevented if care is
taken to treat dry skin early.

Metabolic control

Hyperglycaemia, hypertension, hyperlipidaemia and smoking are the
great quartet of factors that predispose the patient to neuropathy,
ischaemia and, indirectly, via cardiac and kidney impairment, to
swelling of the feet. Thus, good control of blood glucose, blood
pressure, blood cholesterol and triglycerides is extremely important at
Stage 1 to preserve neurological and cardiovascular function.

The results of the Diabetes Control and Complications Trial (DCCT)
and the UK Prospective Diabetes Study demonstrated the value of
good blood glucose control in preventing microvascular complications.
Lowering HbA1C <7% may also reduce the risk of myocardial infarction
and cardiovascular death. Poorly controlled type 1 patients may be
more prone to develop sepsis. To help patients achieve good control
new programmes of diabetes management have been developed.
DAFNE (Dose Adjustment for Normal Eating) is a new programme for
type 1 diabetic patients which enables them to adjust their insulin
dosage to fit in with their lifestyle. DESMOND (Diabetes Education and
Self-Management for Ongoing and Newly Diagnosed) is a new
structured, six hour group education programme for type 2 patients
with an emphasis on self-management and patients setting their own
goals. Both these programmes encourage patients to achieve better

...eful in Stage 1 patients who have problems with

...od pressure is a major risk factor for cardiovascular ...e and microvascular complications and the target should be ...ow 140/80mmHg. In patients with microalbuminuria, the target should be below 130/80mmHg. Angiotensin-converting enzyme inhibitors or Angiotensin-II receptor blockers are first-line therapy for hypertensive patients with microalbuminuria.

Blood lipid control involves lowering low density lipoprotein (LDL) cholesterol, raising high density lipoprotein (HDL) cholesterol and lowering triglycerides. Achieving this reduces macrovascular disease and mortality in patients with type 2 diabetes. Patients should reduce saturated fat and cholesterol intake, and achieve weight loss and increased physical activity levels. (Fig. 2.12). When life-style changes are not successful, statins are first line therapy for hypercholesterolaemia and fibrates for hypertriglyceridaemia. The recent Collaborative-AtoRvastatin Diabetes Study (CARDS) has shown that, compared to placebo, atorvastatin, evoked a significant 37% reduction in the combined primary endpoint of major cardiovascular events in patients with no previous history of cardiovascular disease.

Smoking is a very high risk factor for peripheral vascular disease. Clear unequivocal advice should be given to stop smoking. Enrolment in a smokers' clinic programme may help. All patients with any degree of cardiovascular risk should take daily aspirin.

Hypoglycaemia is a common complication of diabetic treatment and is greatly feared by patients. All health care professionals treating diabetic patients need to know how to diagnose and treat hypoglycaemia. Capillary blood glucose measurement should be available wherever diabetic foot patients are treated, as well as first aid treatment. Warning signs of hypoglycaemia include trembling, paraesthesiae around mouth, shakiness, anxiety, hunger and sweating, confusion, altered behaviour, slurred speech, irritability, drowsiness and, in severe cases, fits and loss of consciousness. If hypoglycaemia is suspected the capillary blood glucose should be measured. A reading below 4mmol confirms hypoglycaemia. If the patient is not drowsy and can swallow, give 130ml Lucozade or 200ml fresh orange juice. On

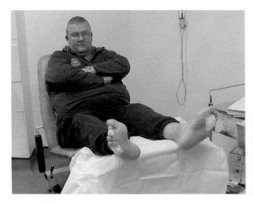

Fig. 2.12
Patient attending diabetic foot clinic with hyperglycaemia, hypertension, hyperlipidaemia and body mass index of 38.

recovery give a slice of bread or two digestive biscuits. If the patient cannot swallow, Hypostop Gel around gums or glucagon 1 mg subcutaneously or intramuscularly (IM) can be given. If very drowsy, give 75ml of 20% glucose intravenously or 1 mg glucagon IM. Hypoglycaemia secondary to sulphonylurea therapy can be prolonged and patients should be admitted and will need intravenous dextrose therapy. Advice on hypoglycaemia prevention should be given.

Educational control

It is easy to teach people the theory of foot care, but extremely difficult to change behaviour. Throughout this book, simple educational material is provided for adaptation and presentation to individual patients and groups (who may include relatives) or to provide topics for workshops or worksheets. Written words need verbal reinforcement and vice versa. Education should be adapted so as to make it relevant for patients of varying ages, backgrounds and cultures. Patients should never be made to feel that they are back in the classroom with an unsympathetic teacher. Patient educators are useful. Frequent educational updating is necessary. Stage 1 patients should be taught about neuropathy and peripheral vascular disease and reassured that good control can delay or prevent complications. They should be taught to expect foot inspection as part of their diabetes annual review.

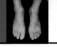
Patient information

SHOES

- Buy well-fitting shoes which fasten with lace or strap
- Look for a foot-shaped shoe
- Shoe heels should be under 5 cm high
- Do not wear slippers all day long.

FOOT CARE

- Wash feet every day and check for problems
- Regular skin care is very important. Apply cream to dry skin. Regular washing should help to prevent skin scales from accumulating
- If problems develop (hard skin, scaly skin, splits, blisters, warts, athletes foot or injuries), seek help from a doctor or podiatrist. Never try to treat the problem yourself, except for simple first aid. Avoid proprietary remedies.

FIRST AID

- Keep a first-aid box at home containing sterile dressings, tape, bandages and antiseptic cream
- If the foot is injured, clean the wound under the tap. Apply antiseptic cream and a bandage or a dressing.

NAILS

- Cut nails after a bath or shower when they are softer
- Do not try to cut the whole nail in one piece
- Do not cut nails too short or leave them poking beyond the end of the toe
- Never cut out the corner of the nail or dig down the sides
- If nails are painful or difficult to cut, then see a state-registered podiatrist. In the UK, treatment is available on the National Health Service.

DAILY FOOT CHECK

- Check feet for danger signs of swelling, colour change, pain or breaks in the skin and seek immediate help if these occur
- Seek advice for minor wounds which do not heal.

Chapter 3

Managing Stage 2: the high-risk foot

PRESENTATION AND DIAGNOSIS

The diabetic foot enters Stage 2 because it has developed one or more of the risk factors for ulceration: neuropathy, ischaemia, deformity, callus and swelling. These may present clinically or else should be detected at annual review.

The foot should be assessed as described in the Introduction and the presence of the above risk factors ascertained. This should be carried out annually so as to detect the onset of risk factors at the earliest opportunity. The foot is then staged and if either neuropathy or ischaemia is present, the foot is classified as neuropathic or neuroischaemic.

Patients with neuropathy or ischaemia are more likely to develop ulceration than patients who have deformity, swelling or callus but have protective pain sensation and an adequate blood supply.

This stage also includes some especially high-risk patients who have previously undergone major or minor amputation (now healed), or have a past history of ulcers, foot infections or necrosis.

MANAGEMENT

The following components of multidisciplinary management are important in Stage 2:

- Mechanical control
- Vascular control
- Metabolic control
- Educational control.

The patient still has intact skin, so wound and microbiological control are irrelevant.

Mechanical control

To maintain mechanical control, deformity and callus must be treated as well as dry skin and fissures secondary to neuropathy. Common

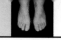

foot problems as described in Stage 1 will also occur and need management as above.

Deformities

Deformities occur in both the neuropathic and neuroischaemic foot. They should be accommodated in properly fitting footwear and may require special bespoke footwear if the deformity is severe. Deformity must not be allowed to precipitate ulceration.

Deformities in the neuropathic foot tend to render the sole vulnerable to ulcers, requiring special insoles, whereas in the neuroischaemic foot, the margins need protection, and appropriately wide shoes should therefore be advised. There should be close liaison between orthotist, podiatrist and physician.

Shoes can be divided into four main types:
- Sensible shoes from the 'high-street' shop
- Ready-made, off-the-shelf, orthopaedic stock shoes which can be extra-depth and/or extra-width (Fig. 3.1). They contain cushioning insoles which are flat non-moulded insoles usually made of microcellular rubber
- Temporary ready-made shoes that can be fitted with cushioning insoles (see Chapter 4)

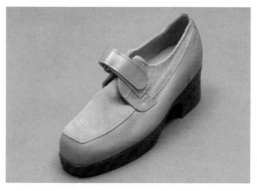

Fig. 3.1
Extra-depth stock shoe.

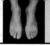

- Customised or bespoke shoes which accommodate the shape of the foot and can house cradled (moulded) insoles which redistribute weight-bearing from vulnerable pressure areas and at the same time provide a suitable cushion (see Chapter 4).

The general principles of shoe prescription are described below.

General principles of shoe prescription
The patient's choice of colour and style should always be respected as far as possible
For young patients, orthopaedic trainers are often acceptable
Patients need shoes for inside and outside, and may need bespoke shoes or boots for work, if steel toe caps are mandatory
Shoes should be reassessed regularly for excessive wear and the changing needs of patients and problems
Patients should have two pairs so that they are never without a pair

Table 3.1
General principles of shoe prescription.

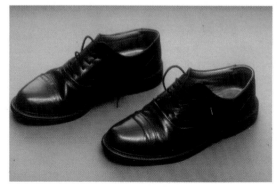

Fig. 3.2
'High-street' shoes with wide toe box.

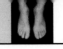
Some deformities may be accommodated in 'high-street' footwear with a wide toe box (Fig. 3.2). Trainer styles are useful. Major deformities which result in red pressure marks on the skin or associated callosities will need either ready-made stock shoes (Fig. 3.1) or bespoke shoes. The more abnormal the foot shape the greater the need for bespoke shoes.

As an alternative to conservative management, prophylactic surgery may sometimes be helpful to correct deformed feet but may be contraindicated in the presence of neuropathy because of the danger of precipitating a Charcot foot. If there is ischaemia, surgery should not be performed. Patients require careful assessment prior to surgery and should be followed carefully throughout the peri-operative and post-operative period. Most of the prophylactic surgical procedures described for the Stage 2 foot can be conducted under local anaesthetic as day cases. The management of specific deformities will now be discussed.

CLAW TOES

CONSERVATIVE MANAGEMENT Claw toes will be susceptible to ulceration on the dorsal surface (Fig. 3.3a) as well as the apex and will need a shoe with a wide, deep, soft toe box to reduce pressure on the dorsum of the toes. This may be obtainable from the 'high-street' shop but it may be necessary to supply extra-depth shoes with a cushioning insole, particularly to protect the apices of the toes (see also Chapter 4). A silicone rubber orthotic can be used to divert pressure from the dorsum of the claw toe (Fig. 3.3b).

SURGICAL MANAGEMENT Arthroplasty can be performed and the position of the toes maintained by means of Kirschner wires.

HAMMER TOES

CONSERVATIVE MANAGEMENT Hammer toes are susceptible to callus formation and ulceration on the dorsum of the toe. A shoe with a wide, deep toe box will help to reduce pressure. Felt padding is useful short-term. Silicone devices can be manufactured to off-load sites of high pressure.

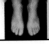

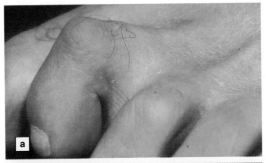

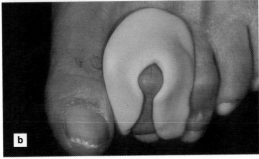

Fig. 3.3
(a) A claw toe.
(b) Silicone rubber orthotic to divert pressure from dorsum of claw toe.

SURGICAL MANAGEMENT If there is fixed deformity a proximal interphalangeal joint arthroplasty can be performed. The extensor tendon is exposed and retracted, the medial and lateral ligaments are freed, and the head of the proximal phalanx is transected. The extensor tendon is repaired and can be lengthened. The new position of the toe can be maintained with a Kirschner wire.

MALLET TOES

CONSERVATIVE MANAGEMENT These may form callus on the dorsum and the apex of the toe. A silicone toe prop or apical crescent may be useful, together with a shoe with a wide, deep toe box.

SURGICAL MANAGEMENT Distal interphalangeal joint arthroplasty corrects mallet toe deformity. The extensor tendon and joint capsule are removed, the collateral ligaments severed and the intermediate phalanx is severed. A Kirschner wire maintains the new position of the joint.

PROMINENT METATARSAL HEADS

CONSERVATIVE MANAGEMENT These are vulnerable on the plantar surface. An extra-depth stock shoe with a cushioning insole may suffice. However, in the presence of a very high arch and extremely prominent metatarsal heads, a cradled insole in bespoke shoes will be needed (see Chapter 4).

SURGICAL MANAGEMENT Surgical management involves resection of one or more metatarsal heads. This is rarely performed except in cases of chronic plantar ulceration or osteomyelitis of the metatarsal head, but may also be useful in patients with intermittent plantar ulceration where it is difficult to maintain healing long-term. The joint is exposed, collateral ligaments cut through, and an oblique cut made in the metatarsal shaft to enable removal of the metatarsal head.

HALLUX RIGIDUS

CONSERVATIVE MANAGEMENT This leads to plantar callus on the first toe. If persistent heavy callus is a problem, then a rocker should be applied to the sole of the shoe by the orthotist to off-load pressure as the foot leaves the ground during the toe-off phase of the gait cycle (Fig. 3.4).

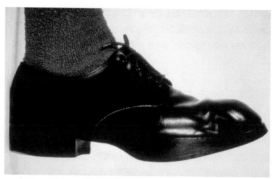

Fig. 3.4
Rocker sole to
relieve pressure
under the hallux.

SURGICAL MANAGEMENT Two surgical options are hallux interphalangeal joint arthroplasty and Keller's resectional arthroplasty of the first metatarso-phalangeal joint. In the latter, more commonly used procedure, the collateral ligaments are severed, the base of the proximal phalanx is removed, and the joint capsule is closed. Kirschner wires can be used to maintain the new position of the toe.

HALLUX VALGUS

CONSERVATIVE MANAGEMENT This common deformity will need a wide toe box to avoid pressure on the medial convexity. This is a common site of ulceration in the neuroischaemic foot and extra-width stock orthopaedic shoes will be often required.

SURGICAL MANAGEMENT Keller's resectional arthroplasty is frequently performed but is unsuitable for young, active patients. An alternative procedure is metatarsal osteotomy.

FIBRO-FATTY PADDING DEPLETION

CONSERVATIVE MANAGEMENT Cushioned insoles, sometimes incorporating silicone or poron inserts, are useful.

SURGICAL MANAGEMENT Injections of silicone are occasionally used to augment fibro-fatty padding to prevent callus formation and subsequent ulceration. Percutaneous lengthening of the Achilles tendon may also be performed to reduce pressure over the plantar forefoot diminishing subsequent callus formation. A triple hemisection technique involves making three percutaneous cuts in the tendon through small stab wounds, following which the position of the foot is corrected and maintained in a plaster cast or brace for several weeks.

Callus

Callus, particularly plantar callus, is a characteristic feature of the neuropathic foot. It also occurs in the neuroischaemic foot but to a much lesser extent. It is the most important preulcerative lesion in Stage 2.

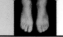

If allowed to become too thick, the callus will press on the soft tissues underneath and cause ulceration. Speckles of blood (Fig. 3.5a) or a deeper layer of whitish, macerated, moist tissue found under the surface of the callus indicate that the foot is close to ulceration and urgent removal of callus is necessary (Fig. 3.5b). Patients should never cut their callus off or use proprietary corn or callus removers. These contain strong acids and allow infection to enter the foot. Instead, the callus should be removed by the podiatrist and regular, sufficiently frequent removal will prevent ulceration.

The easiest way to remove the callus is with a scalpel while ensuring that the fingers of the other hand maintain good skin tension. Sharp debridement should only be performed by experts, as uneven removal can lead to focal points of very high pressure and invasion of the callus by nerve endings and blood vessels which can make future callus removal difficult.

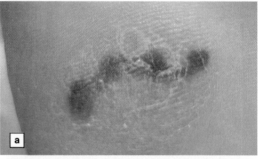

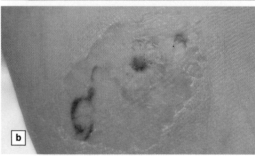

Fig. 3.5
(a) Bleeding under neglected callus.
(b) The same site after callus has been removed by a podiatrist.

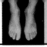

Follow-up is crucial. Patients who fail to keep appointments should be offered a further appointment.

If callus reforms repeatedly, this indicates that there are high pressures acting on the plantar surface of the foot, which need redistribution with footwear before the patient develops ulceration.

An unusual way to remove callus is to have it removed by a pet dog (Fig 3.6).

Dry skin and fissures

Dry skin should be treated with an emollient such as E45 cream or Calmurid cream and the margins of fissures may be reduced with a scalpel. Patients should be encouraged to take great care of their skin on a daily basis.

Common foot problems

Common foot problems may occur in the Stage 2 foot; treatment is described in Chapter 2. All breaks in the skin that are not healing well in 48 hours should be regarded as ulcers and treated as Stage 3. Close observation will be needed especially if ischaemia is present (see Chapter 4). Healing of such lesions will be slow if the foot is swollen.

Partial nail avulsion (PNA) for onychocryptosis is sometimes needed in patients with a degree of ischaemia. The peripheral circulation should be assessed and the feasibility of angioplasty

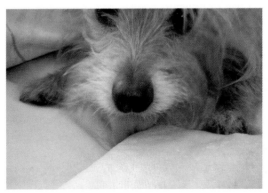

Fig. 3.6
Pet dog chews callus off her owner's feet.

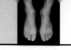

considered to improve the arterial inflow to the foot. PNA should not be carried out as an outpatient procedure in the presence of ischaemia.

Vascular control

Patients with absent foot pulses should have the pressure index measured to confirm ischaemia and to provide a baseline, so that subsequent deterioration can be detected before the patient presents with irreversible lesions. Podiatrists should always ascertain their patient's vascular status before they cut the toe nails or remove callus, since any injury to the neuroischaemic foot can result in ulceration.

All diabetic patients with evidence of peripheral vascular disease may benefit from antiplatelet agents: 75 mg aspirin daily, or if this cannot be tolerated, clopidogrel 75 mg daily.

Diabetic patients with peripheral vascular disease should also be given statin therapy. The Heart Protection Study has shown that simvastatin reduced the rate of major vascular events in a wide range of high-risk patients including those with peripheral arterial disease or diabetes. Patients who are above 55 years and have peripheral vascular disease should also benefit from an angiotensin-converting enzyme inhibitor to prevent further vascular episodes (as indicated by the Heart Outcomes Prevention Evaluation (HOPE) study).

Severe peripheral vascular disease can present as a pink, painful, pulseless foot including the toes (Fig. 3.7), and ulceration is imminent. If the patient has rest pain (persistent pain, secondary to ischaemia and often relieved by letting the foot hang down), disabling claudication or the pressure index is below 0.5, then he already has severe ischaemia and urgent vascular investigations should be carried out.

A sudden occlusion of a major artery, usually popliteal or superficial femoral, will result in a pale, painful, cold foot with purplish mottling. Initially, the skin is intact but if treatment is delayed necrosis will develop and its management is described in Chapter 6.

Patients with claudication alone should enter an exercise programme. Pharmacological treatment is possible with cilostazol, 100mg twice daily.

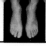

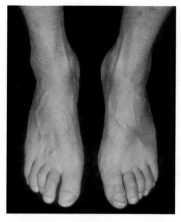

Fig. 3.7
Pink, painful ischaemic foot on·right
compared with well-perfused foot on left.

Metabolic control

Even though neuropathy or ischaemia is now present, progression
may be checked by treating hyperglycaemia, hypertension,
hyperlipidaemia and smoking as described in Chapter 2. Such
treatment may require many different medicines (Fig. 3.8).

Swelling may complicate both the neuropathic and the
neuroischaemic foot. Its main cause will be impaired cardiac and
renal function, which should be assessed and then treated
accordingly. Venous insufficiency can cause swelling and should be
investigated with duplex scanning, treated with compression hose if
there is no peripheral arterial disease and referred for a vascular
opinion. Venous insufficiency may be caused by local venous
disease, but may reflect other conditions which lead to a rise in
venous pressure, including cardiac failure.

Patients in end-stage renal failure treated with haemodialysis may
have variable degrees of oedema and it is important for the footwear
to be adjustable to accommodate fluctuant oedema. Fluctuant
swelling of the stump may be a problem when fitting a patient who
has previously undergone major amputation with a prosthesis.

Neuropathic oedema may respond to ephedrine starting at a
dose of l0 mg t.d.s., but this dose may need to be increased up to
30–60 mg t.d.s.

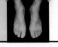

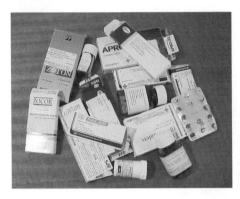

Fig. 3.8
Polytherapy – this patient
needs 14 different drugs to
achieve good metabolic
control.

Educational control

Patients may have lost protective pain sensation and therefore they
need to protect their feet from mechanical, thermal and chemical
trauma. They should compensate for lack of protective pain
sensation by establishing a habit of regular inspection of the feet so
that problems can be detected quickly and help sought sufficiently
early. It is important to educate Stage 2 patients to avoid trauma as
far as possible. Patients who go away on holiday are particularly
prone to develop foot problems and need special advice.

Patient information
FOOT CARE

Your diabetes has made your feet numb. You may not feel pain if
you injure your feet. Please take special precautions to keep your
feet safe.

- Don't walk bare footed
- Visit a podiatrist regularly if you have callus. If you miss an
  appointment, make another quickly
- Never try to remove corns or callus yourself. Corn cures are
  very dangerous if you have diabetes (Fig. 3.9)
- Be careful not to burn your feet (Fig. 3.10). Always check the
  temperature of the bath or shower water with your elbow or use
  a bath thermometer. The water should be below 45°C. Never

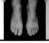

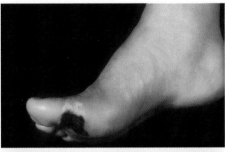

Fig. 3.9
Necrosis of first toe
following application of corn
cure.

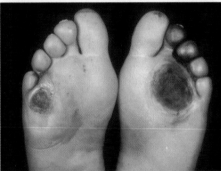

Fig. 3.10
Burns to feet from placing
them in very hot water.

apply direct heat to your feet. Switch off electric blankets and
remove hot water bottles before going to bed
- Position your bed away from wall radiators and hot water pipes
- Never toast your toes in front of the fire
- Prevent dryness in your feet by using a moisture-restoring
  cream
- If problems develop (splits, blisters, warts, athletes foot or
  injuries), seek help. Never try to treat the problem yourself,
  except for simple first-aid.

FOOTWEAR

- Shake out any loose pebbles or grit that may have found its way
  into the shoes before you put them on

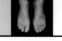
- Run a hand around the insides of the shoes to detect rough, worn places
- If the hospital gives you shoes, please wear them all the time that you are on your feet
- If your shoes are wearing out, get them repaired or replaced in plenty of time. If shoe problems develop, seek help.

DANGER SIGNS Check your feet every day for:
- Colour change
- Pain or discomfort
- Breaks in the skin or discharge
- Swelling
- Callus.

HOLIDAY FOOT-CARE EDUCATION

THE JOURNEY
- Wear shoes with adjustable fastening to accommodate swelling
- Arrange a wheelchair if you have foot problems
- Allow plenty of time for your journey
- If in a car or coach, take frequent stops to stretch your legs.

FLYING
- Allow plenty of time at the airport
- Don't carry heavy luggage: use a trolley
- Arrange a wheelchair if you have foot problems
- Ask for an aisle seat – walk up and down every half hour to prevent swelling
- Do not get dehydrated – keep sipping water
- Wear shoes with adjustable fastenings
- Beware of trolleys pushed by other passengers in a hurry.

ON ARRIVAL
- Hot sand and sharp rocks or broken glass can cause serious injuries. Wear plastic sandals on the beach and in the sea
- Use sun block or very high factor sunscreen or keep in the shade

- Apply cream to dry skin. Calmurid is very effective for this if normal creams do not help.

FIRST AID

- Take a small first-aid kit on holiday containing plasters, sterile dressings, bandage, tape and antiseptic cream
- Clean and cover all injuries, however slight
- Check them daily. Seek help if they get worse.

HOLIDAY FOOTWEAR

- Never wear new shoes on holiday. They may cause rubs
- If you have hospital shoes, continue to wear them on holiday
- Wear hose to prevent blisters.

IN SUBTROPICAL OR TROPICAL COUNTRIES

- Backpackers with neuropathy should beware of rats. One of the authors' sons was woken in India by a rat nibbling his toes
- Use insect repellant and mosquito netting to avoid insect bites or stings.

Chapter 4

Managing Stage 3: the ulcerated foot

PRESENTATION AND DIAGNOSIS

This is the stage of skin breakdown and ulceration. Every break of the skin in the diabetic foot is a portal of entry for bacteria and has the potential for disaster. We have seen patients who came to a major amputation following a trivial lesion. A diabetic foot lesion should never be regarded as trivial. After initial diagnosis, early aggressive treatment should be instituted and the patient followed up until it is healed and has remained healed for at least a month.

A classification of ulcers has not been attempted, as it is necessary to assess each ulcer on its own merits and then plan a specific treatment. Ulceration can present in many ways but it is essential to differentiate between ulceration in the neuropathic foot compared with that in the neuroischaemic foot. Furthermore, it is important to diagnose special categories of ulcers including:

- Decubitus ulcer
- Puncture wound
- Chemical and thermal traumatic wound
- Iatrogenic ulcer
- Artifactual ulcer
- Malignant ulcer
- Ulcer overlying the Achilles tendon.

It is advisable to X-ray feet with newly presenting ulcers to detect:

- Loss of bone density or cortical destruction, suggesting osteomyelitis
- Foreign body
- Gas in the deep tissues, indicating severe infection
- Charcot osteoarthropathy.

Neuropathic ulcer

The neuropathic ulcer is usually painless, and the commonest site is the apex of the toe, which when associated with a claw toe

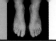

deformity, develops callus on a plantar pressure site, and then breaks down (Fig. 4.1).

Callus forms over the dorsal aspect of the toes due to the pressure of footwear on the flexed interphalangeal joint. Callus also develops on the plantar aspect of prominent metatarsal heads, often associated with fibro-fatty padding depletion, and failure to remove the callus leads to ulceration (Figs. 4.2a and b). Removal of callus

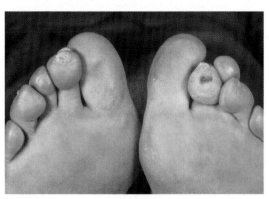

Fig. 4.1
Ulcer at the apex of a clawed second toe. The apex of the second toe on the contralateral foot shows neglected callus.

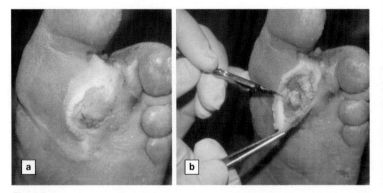

Fig. 4.2
(a) Callus over the forefoot has been left too long as it was not painful.
(b) Debridement by the podiatrist reveals tissue breakdown – the birth of a neuropathic ulcer.

may often reveal ulcers (Figs. 4.3a and b). Ulcers on the plantar aspect of the heel are usually caused by acute trauma, in particular, treading on foreign bodies.

On initial observation, a neuropathic ulcer may seem shallow. It is always important to probe an ulcer, as this may reveal hidden depths (Figs. 4.4a and b), and also reveal a sinus down to bone suggesting osteomyelitis.

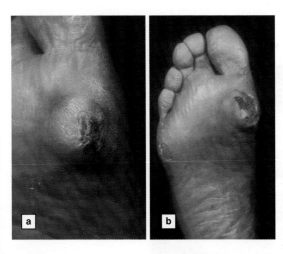

Fig. 4.3
(a) Heavy callus overlying neuropathic ulcer. (b) Callus has been removed to reveal neuropathic ulcer.

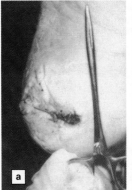
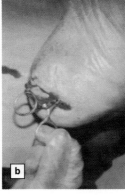

Fig. 4.4
(a) An apparently shallow ulcer and a pair of 6-cm artery forceps. (b) Probing the ulcer reveals its true extent as the forceps tracks through the subcutaneous tissues.

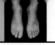

Neuroischaemic ulcer

Ulceration in the neuroischaemic foot usually occurs on the margins of the foot. The first sign of ischaemic ulceration is a red mark which blisters (Fig. 4.5) and then develops into a shallow ulcer with a base of sparse pale granulations or yellowish closely adherent slough. In ischaemia there is often a halo of erythema around the ulcer (Fig. 4.6).

Although ulcers occur on the medial surface of the first metatarso-phalangeal joint (particularly if hallux valgus is present), and over the lateral aspect of the fifth metatarso-phalangeal joint, the commonest sites are the apices of the toes (Fig. 4.7) and also beneath any toe nails if allowed to become overly thick (Fig. 4.8).

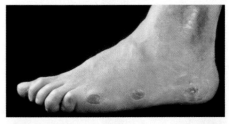

Fig. 4.5
New ischaemic ulcers resulting from blisters on lateral margin of foot.

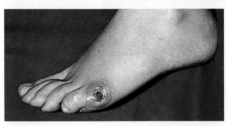

Fig. 4.6
An ischaemic ulcer on the margin of the foot with a halo of erythema

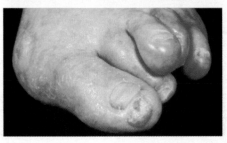

Fig. 4.7
Ischaemic ulceration on apex of the first toe.

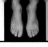

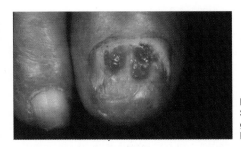

Fig. 4.8
Subungual ulcer. The nail had grown too thick. It is cut back to reveal the ulcer.

Decubitus ulcer

All patients with neuropathic or neuroischaemic feet are at risk of decubitus ulcers. These may develop after a period of illness or immobilisation or after a severe hypoglycaemic episode, on the trolley in casualty, on the ward or even on the operating table, and the heels are particularly vulnerable sites.

The first sign of a heel sore is localized erythema. If pressure is not relieved, a blister develops which fills with serosanguinous fluid. The base of the blister becomes blue and then black. If pressure remains unrelieved, necrosis may develop.

Puncture wound

These may appear as pinpoint injuries usually caused by a foreign body which may have inoculated bacteria at the base of the injury. There is often no direct evidence of deep tissue damage, and infection will only become manifest when it has tracked back to the surface. A foreign body can be detected by X-ray if radio-opaque. Otherwise, ultrasound can be used.

Chemical and thermal traumatic wound

Chemical trauma may originate from proprietary remedies including corn cure and callus removers which contain strong acids and undiluted antiseptics applied directly to wounds

Thermal traumas include burns from hot baths or showers, hot water bottles and electric blankets, hot sand on beaches, poultices, fires and radiators. Patients are also susceptible to cold trauma.

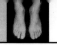
Frostbite in diabetic patients who stay outside in wintry conditions (one patient worked in a meat market and stayed in a walk-in deep freezer for too long) can cause severe tissue damage.

Dog, cat and rat bites and scratches, bee and wasp stings and insect bites can all cause ulceration.

Iatrogenic ulcer

Iatrogenic ulcers are caused by tape applied to atrophic skin and ripped off, by over-tight bandages and by bulky dressings which are not accommodated in roomy footwear. We have seen ulcers caused by capillary blood samples which were taken from the toe instead of the finger and severe and indolent ulceration following cortisone injections into the heel.

Artifactual ulcer

Perhaps saddest of all, a very small minority of patients deliberately cause ulcers and prevent them from healing (Fig. 4.9). Some diabetic patients appear to traumatise their feet deliberately to cause ulceration and then prevent the resulting wound from healing. Most patients are young and female and may have a history of 'brittle diabetes' or eating disorders.

Malignant ulcer

Any pigmented lesion which enlarges, develops satellite lesions or an irregular edge, erosions or ulceration may be a malignant

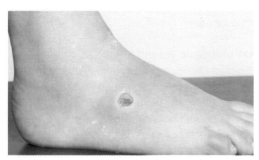

Fig. 4.9
Artifactual ulcer caused by application of lavatory cleaner.

melanoma and should be seen urgently by a dermatologist. Some melanomas are not associated with pigment (Fig. 4.10). Squamous cell carcinoma may occasionally masquerade as an indolent diabetic foot ulcer (Figs. 4.11a and b).

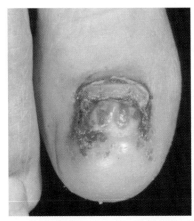

Fig. 4.10
Amelanotic malignant melanoma, which is not pigmented.

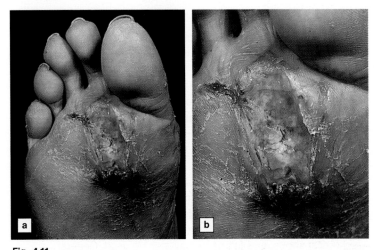

Fig. 4.11
(a) Ulcer following application of a proprietary wart remedy which proved to be a squamous cell carcinoma. (b) Close-up of lesion.

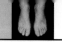

Ulcer overlying the Achilles tendon

This is a notoriously difficult site to heal. Ulceration is usually triggered by unsuitable footwear or is a pressure lesion in an immobile patient. When tendon is exposed in the base of the ulcer then this may need to be surgically removed. Hyaff (hyaluronic acid ester dressing) (see page 81) may encourage granulation over healthy tendon.

MANAGEMENT

All of the components of multidisciplinary management are important in Stage 3:

- Mechanical control
- Wound control
- Microbiological control
- Vascular control
- Metabolic control
- Educational control.

The aim is to heal ulcers within the first six weeks of their development. This is the time for early and aggressive management and is a window of opportunity that should be taken seriously.

Mechanical control

Ideally, ulcers must be managed with rest and avoidance of pressure. However, total non-weight bearing is rarely practical and ambulatory methods have been developed.

In the neuropathic foot the overall aim is to redistribute plantar pressures, while in the neuroischaemic foot it is to protect the vulnerable margins of the foot. Thus, mechanical control will be considered separately in the neuropathic and neuroischaemic foot.

Neuropathic foot

The most efficient way to redistribute plantar pressure is by the immediate application of some form of cast. If casting techniques are not available, temporary ready-made shoes with a cushioning insole can be supplied. These can take the form of dressing shoes or weight-relief shoes, and felt pads may also be used. General

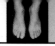

measures such as the use of crutches, wheelchairs and Zimmer frames should be encouraged.

Heel ulcers will need specific off-loading techniques such as a foam wedge or a pressure relief ankle foot orthosis (PRAFO).

When the neuropathic ulcer has healed, the patient should be fitted with a cradled insole and bespoke shoes to prevent recurrence. Occasionally, extra-depth, ready-made orthopaedic shoes with flat cushioning insoles may suffice in the absence of very high pressure areas.

Casts

Various casts are available and their use is governed by local experience and expertise. Techniques include the removable cast walker such as Aircast, the total contact cast and the Scotchcast boot,

Removable cast walker

Prefabricated walking casts have become popular because of the potential problems with total contact casts, as described below. The Aircast (Fig. 4.12) is a bivalved cast and the halves are joined together with velcro strapping. The Aircast is lined with four air cells which can be inflated with a hand pump through four valves to ensure a

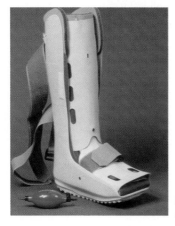

Fig. 4.12
Aircast.

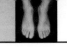

close fit. Care must be taken that the brace does not impinge on the borders of the foot. It is removable so patients can check their ulcers and remove the cast in bed. However, this very fact which makes the cast seem potentially safe renders it unsuitable for some patients who may find it difficult to wear the cast continuously and use it only intermittently. Aircast can be simply adapted with a heat gun applied to the outer shell, which is then softened and bent out to accommodate deformity. Felt padding may be stuck on to the lining of the Aircast to off-load discrete areas. The Aircast is supplied with flat-bed insoles which can be replaced by cradled insoles. It is available in small, medium, large and extra large sizes. The Aircast is removable, but can be rendered irremovable (the "Instant Total Contact Cast") by wrapping fibreglass tape around it, and this technique can be applied to other removable walking braces.

TOTAL CONTACT CAST

This is the treatment of choice for indolent neuropathic ulcers and acute Charcot osteoarthropathy. It is a very efficient method of redistributing plantar pressure. However, it is not without its complications and should be reserved for plantar ulcers that have not responded to other casting treatments. It is a close-fitting Plaster of Paris and fibreglass cast applied over minimum padding (Fig. 4.13). It enforces compliance as the patient cannot remove it.

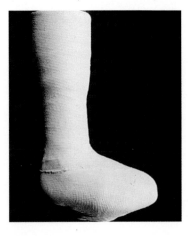

Fig. 4.13
The total contact cast.

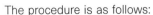

The procedure is as follows:

- A layer of stockinette should be applied to the patient's lower leg. The length of the stockinette should be twice the distance from knee to toes and the excess should be gathered up over the knee and later folded down over the cast to cover any roughness. Cast padding is placed between the toes to prevent rubs. The distal end of the stockinette is closed with tape and any creases in the stockinette are cut out and taped flat
- Seven millimetres thick pieces of adhesive felt are applied over bony prominences including medial and lateral malleoli, tibial crest (and a prominent tuberosity of the navicular or styloid process)
- A thin layer of cast padding is applied to the entire below the knee area, with thicker layers at the proximal end of the cast and the area over the toes as these are the areas where rubs most frequently occur
- Plaster of Paris bandage is wrapped around the foot and leg starting 3 cm below the cast padding and rubbed gently on to the contours and then reinforced with several layers of fibreglass tape. Many practitioners omit Plaster of Paris altogether and use only fibreglass tape which is a simpler and less messy procedure and obviates the need for a plaster trap on the clinic sink
- The excess stockinette (which was gathered up over the knee at the beginning of the procedure) and the proximal 3 cm of cast padding are pulled down and over the cast and provide a smooth finish
- If the cast is applied to the neuropathic foot with a post-operative wound, it may be necessary to cut a window in the cast at the site of the wound in order to observe it closely.

Common mistakes are to make the cast too lightweight, to handle and rub the Plaster of Paris bandage with the finger tips instead of the flat of the hands, or to apply the cast to a plantar-flexed foot.

Practitioners should never attempt to apply a cast simply after reading a description or seeing photographs of the technique. Applying casts is technically demanding and training and experience are needed. If possible, the hospital plaster room should be involved.

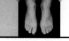

The plaster technicians should be asked to make all casts stronger and heavier than for a patient with normal sensation and the outside of the cast should always be covered with stockinette to prevent scratches on the other leg.

It is dangerous to enclose an insensitive foot in a closed cast without careful education of the patient. Patients should monitor their temperature and blood glucose daily.

The instructions given to our patients are shown in Table 4.1. Patients in total contact casts should not fly because of the danger of developing deep vein thrombosis.

Casts should be initially removed after one week for wound inspection. They should be then renewed and removed at regular intervals. Once the ulcer is healed, the patient should be assessed for cradled insoles and bespoke shoes. He should remain in the total contact cast until the new shoes are ready. He will then be ready for

Instructions for patients
Ring immediately:
If your temperature rises above 37.5 °C
If your blood glucose rises above 15 mmol/L
If you feel unwell, tired, hot, shivery, with flu-like symptoms
If you feel pain or discomfort in your foot or leg
If your cast becomes loose, tight, stained, wet, soft, cracked or smelling badly
Never poke or pour anything down your cast
Never try to remove your cast yourself
Walk as little as possible

Table 4.1
Instructions for patients fitted with a total contact cast.

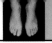

rehabilitation as follows:

- a removable, bivalved cast should be made by cutting out the front of the total contact cast and then holding the two halves in place with a bandage or Velcro strapping. However, the removable bi-valved cast is less efficient than the total contact cast, and putting the patient into an Aircast may be preferable to bivalving
- the patient may walk for a few steps each day in his new shoes and insoles around the house, but the rest of the time he should wear the removable cast
- very gradually he can build up the amount of time he spends in the shoes and decrease the time spent in the cast
- if blistering or ulceration occur, he should return to the clinic at once
- he should ideally receive rehabilitation from the physiotherapist to build up wasted muscles.

Problems with casts are shown in Table 4.2.

Problems with casts
Risk of iatrogenic lesions (rubs, pressure sores, infections) which may be undetected
Cast often heavy and uncomfortable and reduces patient's mobility
Problems with knee, hip and spine due to leg length disparity. This can be prevented with a shoe raise on the contralateral side
Patient may not drive a car in a cast
The leg may develop immobilization osteoporosis
Danger of fracture and the development of a Charcot foot when coming out of a cast if patient walks too far too soon
A few patients develop a cast phobia and will not wear them. One of our patients borrowed the neighbour's Black and Decker electric saw and removed her cast (but fortunately not her leg)!

Table 4.2
Problems with casts.

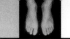

SCOTCHCAST BOOT

This is a simple removable boot made of stockinette, felt and fibreglass tape which is effective in redistributing plantar pressure (Fig. 4.14) A large sock worn over the cast offers some protection to the toes. It is possible to make a version which cannot be taken off if non-compliance is a problem. It is useful for patients with neuroischaemic feet or cast phobia.

The procedure is as follows:

- A layer of stockinette is applied to the lower limb from mid-calf to 10 cm distal to the toes
- 7mm felt is applied to the sole of the foot extending to the tips of the toes, up the back of the heel and up each side of the foot
- Cast padding is wrapped around the foot over the felt
- Overlapping strips of fibreglass tape cover the sole of the foot, and more fibreglass tape is wrapped around the foot
- Fibreglass is trimmed away below the malleoli, round the back of the heel and along the sides of the foot. The fibreglass covering the dorsum of the foot is lifted away
- The stockinette is folded back over the foot from both ends and the entire foot is wrapped in Elastoplast tape
- If a removable boot is required, the dorsal area is cut open, the raw edges are sealed with elastoplast, a strip of felt is used as a protective tongue and the boot is held on with ready-made straps or Velcro fastening.

TEMPORARY SHOES

When it is not possible to provide a cast, ready-made temporary shoes with cushioning insoles that can accommodate dressings or weight-relief shoes may be helpful.

DRESSING SHOES

The Darco boot provides closed toe protection and room for bulky dressings. It can also be fitted with a cushioning insole. The Dru shoe is a Plastazote shoe which has removable Plastazote insoles.

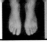

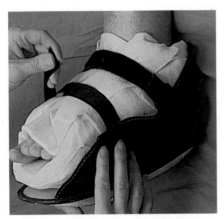

Fig. 4.14
The Scotchcast boot.

WEIGHT-RELIEF SHOES

These take various forms according to the area of the foot which is off-loaded.

- The OrthoWedge shoe off-loads pressure from the metatarsal head and toes using a rocker-bottom wedge design
- The Forefoot relief shoe transfers weight from forefoot to hindfoot with 10 degrees of dorsiflexion built into the shoe. A semi-rigid heel counter provides stability
- The Heel relief shoe eliminates weight bearing on the posterior end of the foot, which is put into a plantar-flex mode to facilitate off- loading of the heel area. Weight is transferred from heel to midfoot and forefoot.

FELT PADDING

Semi-compressed adhesive felt padding is often used to divert pressures from ulcers but can prevent complications from being detected unless lifted regularly.

CRUTCHES

Young and active patients with neuropathic ulcers may do well with crutches. However, patients with postural hypotension may be unsteady. Patients with neuropathy of the hands or Dupuytren's contracture may find hand-held crutches difficult to manage.

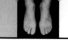

Untrained patients can risk falls especially on stairs, so crutches should always be fitted by a physiotherapist.

WHEELCHAIRS

A light-weight folding wheelchair can be of great help in achieving maximal off-loading. The British Red Cross hires out wheelchairs for a nominal sum (these are not self-propelling).

ZIMMER FRAMES

Many patients who cannot cope with crutches find that a Zimmer frame is more helpful, being light-weight and providing more stability. A simple adaptation of the Zimmer frame uses bent copper tubing to support a cushioned plywood shelf to rest the knee on the ulcerated side so as to ensure that the foot is kept off the ground (Fig. 4.15).

ELECTRIC CARTS AND BUGGIES

Small electrically-powered carts and buggies with rechargeable

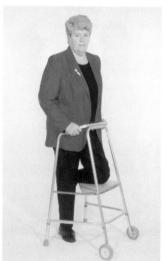

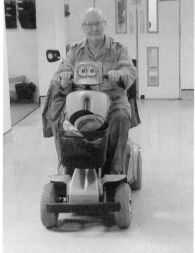

Fig. 4.15
Adapted Zimmer frame. Kneeling on the shelf off-loads the ulcerated foot.

Fig. 4.16
Small electric carts are useful off-loading devices.

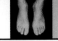

batteries are used by diabetic foot patients with great success
(Fig. 4.16).

CRADLED (OR MOULDED) INSOLES

These are designed to redistribute weight bearing away from the
vulnerable pressure areas and at the same time provide a suitable
cushioning. These insoles often need to be accommodated in
bespoke shoes.

To make a cradled insole, a plaster cast is taken of the foot to
represent its overall contours including the sole. The cast is filled
with a foam to make a last, over which the insoles are moulded, and
shoes constructed. An extra-depth orthopaedic stock shoe can
sometimes accommodate a bespoke insole if the foot itself has a
reasonably normal shape.

A variety of polyethylene foams, microcellular rubbers and ethyl
vinyl acetates are used to construct cradled or moulded insoles,
which are usually made of two or three layers of differing densities,
with the most compressible layer at the foot–insole interface.

MATERIALS
Closed cell polyethylene foam, e.g. Plastazote
- Easily mouldable
- Cushions
- Bottoms out.

Open cell polyurethane rubber e.g. Poron or closed cell synthetic
rubber e.g. Neoprene:
- Not mouldable
- Excellent shock absorption
- Good long-term resilience, will not bottom out
- Firm density.

Ethyl–vinyl–acetate (EVA) e.g. Nora or Evalon range of different
densities of EVAs
- Mouldable
- Resilient
- Elastic.

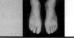

Various designs of cradled or moulded insoles are in use.

EVA insoles have a top layer of low-density EVA for cushioning, followed by two to four layers of medium-density EVA and a base layer of high-density EVA, the most dense and rigid layer acting as a cradle. Under particularly high pressure regions, areas of the insole can be excavated to form a "sink" which is filled in with pressure-relieving material (Fig. 4.17).

The Tovey insole uses a high-density Plastazote material for the cradle. Pressure areas are marked on this and these areas are cut away to be filled in with Neoprene cushioning. The insole is covered with an upper layer of Neoprene cushioning.

Alternatively, composite insoles can be made with an upper layer of low-density Plastazote and a lower layer of polyurethane rubber. Discrete areas of very high pressure can be compensated by insertion of 'sinks' of Poron into the Plastazote.

Neuroischaemic foot

Ulcers in neuroischaemic feet usually develop around the margins of the foot. Many of these lesions are caused by tight shoes or a slip-on style shoe which leads to frictional forces on the vulnerable margins of the foot. A 'high-street' shoe that is sufficiently long, broad and deep and fastens with a lace or strap high on the foot may be all that is needed to control neuroischaemic ulceration.

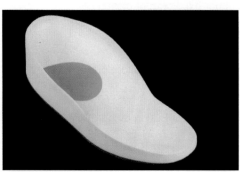

Fig. 4.17
Cradled insole with excavated sink filled with Neoprene to accommodate plantar deformity.

Alternatively, a ready-made stock shoe which is wide-fitting may be suitable. In the first instance, a temporary shoe such as a Darco boot may be used if dressings are bulky. Following healing, an extra-width orthopaedic stock shoe may be worn. Crutches and Zimmer frames may be useful for the neuroischaemic patient as described above for the neuropathic patient.

Surgery as part of mechanical control

Surgery may help to achieve mechanical control by correction of deformity and decompression or excision of ulcers (see below). The potential dangers of surgery on the ischaemic foot and possibility of triggering Charcot osteoarthropathy in the neuropathic foot were mentioned in the previous chapter and also apply to the stage 3 foot. The following techniques are available:

- Ulcer decompression and excision is a possible alternative to conservative pressure-relieving therapy. When indolent neuropathic ulceration develops over an underlying bony prominence, removal of bone and excision of the ulcer may enable the edges of the fresh surgical wound to be approximated. When this is not possible, local random flaps may be used or the wound left to heal by secondary intention
- Procedures already discussed for correction of hammer toe, mallet toe, claw toe, metatarsal head resection and Achilles tendon lengthening can also be used to heal or prevent recurrence of ulcers
- Metatarsal head resection may be useful when underlying osteomyelitis is present. Achilles tendon lengthening may relieve pressure over the forefoot
- Partial calcanectomy is useful when calcaneal bone protrudes from a heel ulcer.

Further details of these operations are described in the companion volume to this book: A Practical Manual of Diabetic Foot Care (Blackwell Science, 2004).

Wound control

Wound control in the neuropathic and neuroischaemic ulcer is centred upon sharp debridement.

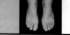

Debridement

NEUROPATHIC ULCER

Debridement is the most important part of wound control. The rationale is described in Table 4.3 and the procedure is as follows:

- Remove all callus surrounding ulcer with a sterile scalpel
- Cut away all slough and non-viable tissue. It is helpful to grip the material to be cut with a pair of forceps and to apply gentle traction so that the material is under tension (Fig. 4.18), while it is being cut. It is almost impossible to remove moist slough with a scalpel blade unless this manoeuvre is performed. Dry gauze may be directly applied to moist slough to remove moisture and thus render it easier to grip. The forceps are also useful for probing an ulcer to ensure its true dimensions
- Probe ulcer (if probe reaches bone, this is indicative of osteomyelitis – regard as Stage 4 foot)
- Take deep swab and tissue samples (not surface callus) and send for culture without delay
- Clean ulcer with sterile normal saline
- Apply sterile dressing held in place with light bandage – not too tight. Tubular bandage is useful
- Review at weekly intervals and repeat the procedure (but ensure the patient knows that if problems develop he should return to clinic immediately).

Rationale for debridement of neuropathic ulcers
Debridement removes callus, thus lowering plantar pressures
It enables the true dimensions of the ulcer to be perceived
Drainage of exudate and removal of dead tissue renders infection less likely
Debridement enables a deep swab to be taken for culture
Debridement encourages healing, restoring a chronic wound to an acute wound

Table 4.3
Rationale for the debridement of neuropathic ulcers.

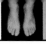

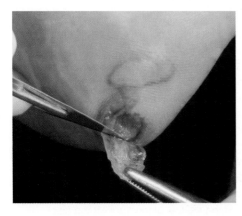

Fig. 4.18
'Scalpel and forceps'
debridement technique.

Outpatient debridement should be regarded as a minor surgical procedure and take place ideally in hospital or clinic. Control of cross-infection is important.

- Pre-prepared sterile packs are useful for ulcer clinics: they contain a disposable instrument tray, sterile field, scalpel handle, blunt forceps and scissors. The contents of the packs are laid out on the top shelf of a two-storey trolley and sterile scalpel blades, dressings, saline, and any other necessary materials are added as needed
- The bottom shelf of the trolley has dressings, conforming bandages, saline ampoules, tubular bandage and hypoallergenic tape. When the patient has left the clinical area, the patient's chair and trolley are cleaned with isopropyl alcohol wipes.

When a neuropathic ulcer has been present for more than 3 months without healing, despite regular debridement and good management, and where bone is exposed in the base of the ulcer, then surgical resection of underlying bone is probably the best way to achieve rapid healing.

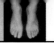

NEUROISCHAEMIC ULCER

The rationale for debridement is described in Table 4.4, and the procedure is as follows:

- Vascular status should be quantified by measuring the pressure index before debridement. Only very cautious debridement should be performed if the foot is very ischaemic (pressure index <0.5)
- Some ischaemic ulcers develop a halo of thin glassy callus which dries out, becomes hard and curls up. (Figs. 4.19a and b). It is necessary to smooth off these areas as they can catch on dressings and cause trauma to underlying tissue
- If the foot is very sensitive, it may be necessary to anchor the area being debrided with forceps while cutting takes place so as not to cause painful dragging of the scalpel blade through the slack tissues
- If a subungual ulcer beneath a thickened toe nail is suspected, the nail should be very gently cut back or layers of nail can be pared away with a scalpel, to expose and drain the ulcer
- It is very unwise to inject local anaesthetic into an ischaemic foot.

Supplementary techniques of wound control
MAGGOTS (LARVATHERAPY).

The larvae of the green bottle fly (which feed on dead flesh) are sometimes used to debride ulcers, especially in the neuroischaemic foot. Only sterile maggots obtained from a medical maggot farm should be used (Fig 4.20).

Rationale for debridement of neuroischaemic ulcers
It enables the true dimensions of the ulcer to be perceived
Drainage of exudate and removal of dead tissue renders infection less likely
Debridement enables a deep swab to be taken for culture

Table 4.4
Rationale for debridement of neuroischaemic ulcers.

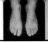

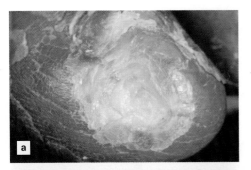

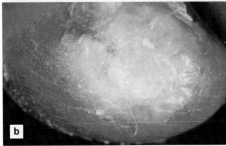

Fig. 4.19
(a) An ischaemic ulcer with halo of thin glassy callus. (b) The halo has been cut away without causing trauma.

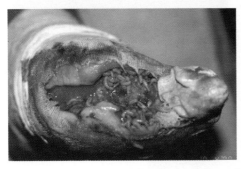

Fig. 4.20
Maggots in wound.

SKIN GRAFT

To speed healing of ulcers which have a clean granulating wound bed, a split skin graft may be harvested and applied to the ulcer. If chosen from within the distribution of sensory neuropathy, the donor site will be less painful.

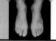
VACUUM-ASSISTED CLOSURE

The vacuum-assisted closure (VAC) pump is used to achieve closure of wounds, including diabetic foot wounds (Figs 4.21a,b,c,d,e). It is important to use the pump on wounds that have been thoroughly debrided and do not contain slough. The pump applies continuous negative pressure of 125mmHg to the ulcer through a tube and foam sponge which are applied to the ulcer and sealed in place with a

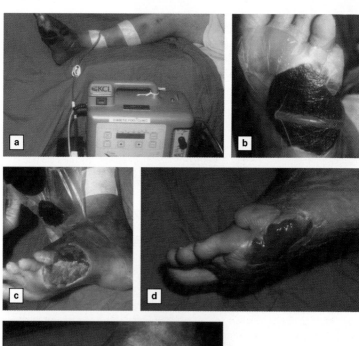

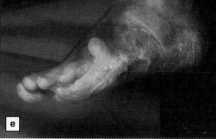

Fig. 4.21
(a) VAC pump attached to patient's foot. (b) Sponge attached to plantar aspect of foot. (c) Sponge being removed from the foot. (d) Ulcer healing after 10 days VAC therapy. (e) Ulcer healed.

plastic film to create a vacuum. The sponge is replaced every two or three days. Exudate from the wound is sucked along the tube to a disposable collecting chamber. The negative pressure improves the dermal blood supply, and stimulates granulation which can form even over bone and tendon. It reduces bacterial colonization and diminishes oedema and interstitial fluid. Recently, installation tubes have been added to the pump to facilitate application of topical antibiotics. The VAC pump is increasingly used to treat post-operative wounds in the diabetic ischaemic foot especially when revascularization is not possible (see page 118).

Hyperbaric oxygen

Studies involving relatively small groups of patients have shown that hyperbaric oxygen accelerates the healing of ischaemic diabetic foot ulcers. Adjunctive systemic hyperbaric oxygen therapy has been shown to reduce the number of major amputations in ischaemic diabetic feet. It is reasonable to use hyberbaric oxygen as an adjunctive in severe or life threatening wounds.

Dressings

Sterile, non-adherent dressings should cover all open diabetic foot lesions to protect them from trauma, absorb exudate, reduce infection and promote healing. There is no hard evidence from large studies that any dressing is better or worse than any other. However, the following dressing properties are essential for the diabetic foot: ease and speed of lifting, ability to be walked on without disintegrating and good exudate control.

Dressings should be lifted every day to ensure that problems or complications are detected quickly, especially in patients who lack protective pain sensation. The types of dressings used in diabetic foot patients and their relevant features are described below.

Foams

- Very absorbent
- Bulky – may need specially roomy shoe to accommodate
- Conforms to contours
- Cushioning effect.

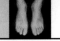

ALGINATES
- Only to be used on moist exuding wounds
- High absorbency
- Drying out of dressing may prevent wound drainage
- Calcium alginate is a good haemostatic agent.

HYDROGELS
- Promote autolysis and therefore promote debridement
- May cause maceration
- Risk of changing dry necrosis into wet necrosis.

HYDROPHILIC FIBRE DRESSINGS
- Non-adherent
- Absorbent
- Conform to the wound.

HYDROCOLLOIDS
- Designed to be left on for several days
- Daily changing prevents dressing from acting optimally
- Can be used only in patients with protective pain sensation
- Patient can bathe and shower.

SILVER-IMPREGNATED DRESSINGS
- Releases silver ions
- Antimicrobial actions
- Useful in exudating wound which may have early infection

KERRABOOT
- New transparent device in the form of a boot (Fig. 4.22)
- Enables easy inspection of the ulcer and lower limb
- Easy removal
- Rapid re-dressing.

OTHER DRESSINGS
- Simple non-adherent dressings are useful and nontraumatic
- Saline soaked gauze is widely used throughout the world.

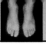

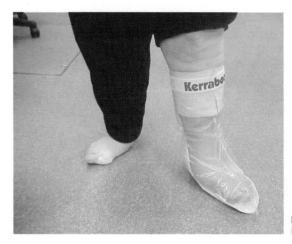

Fig. 4.22
Kerraboot.

FASTENING DRESSINGS

Hypoallergenic tape and tubular bandages are useful. Only small amounts of tape should be applied to the skin. Encircling the entire toe with tape should be avoided in case it swells.

Topical therapy

This consists of cleansing agents and antimicrobials.

CLEANSING AGENTS

SALINE

We use saline as a wound cleansing agent. It does not interfere with microbiological samples and is not damaging to granulating tissue.

ANTIMICROBIALS

IODINE

Iodine is effective against a wide spectrum of organisms and comes in a variety of formulations including solutions, alcoholic tinctures, powder sprays and impregnated dressings. At high concentrations it can be toxic to human cells but bacteria are more sensitive to these effects than human cells such as fibroblasts, and thus it is believed that iodine may be useful for antisepsis without impairing wound

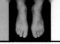

healing. At present two types of iodine are available, Povidone-iodine and Cadexomer iodine. Povidone-iodine is effective in anti-bacterial prophylaxis in burn patients but evidence of its efficacy in other wound types is awaited. Cadexomer iodine consists of microspheres formed from a three-dimensional lattice of cross-linked starch chains (cadexomers) and has been used with success in the diabetic foot ulcer.

Silver compounds
Silver sulphadiazine has been used in antibacterial prophylaxis in wounds and in skin graft donor sites. It is possible that silver may be useful as prophylaxis in diabetic foot ulcers. In vitro it is effective in killing staphylococcus aureus, including methicillin resistant staphylococcus aureus, and pseudomonas species.

Mupirocin
Mupirocin is active against Gram-positive bacteria including MRSA. To avoid the development of resistance, mupirocin should not be used for longer than ten days and should not be regarded as a prophylactic.

Advanced Wound-Healing Products
These include:
- Dermagraft
- Apligraf
- Platelet-derived growth factor (Regranex)
- Protease inhibitors
- Hyaluronic acid ester.

Dermagraft is a bioengineered living human dermis, which is delivered frozen but needs to be thawed, warmed and rinsed prior to application. Controlled trials have shown significant improvement in neuropathic ulcers treated with Dermagraft.

Apligraf is a bioengineered, bilayered, skin substitute consisting of human fibroblasts embedded in bovine collagen and covered by human keratinocytes. It is stored in an incubator. Controlled studies have shown significantly increased healing rates in neuropathic ulcers.

Platelet-derived growth factor (Regranex) stimulates chemotaxis and mitogenesis of neutrophils, fibroblasts and monocytes. It is used in the form of a gel and several trials have shown significantly improved healing rates compared with controls.

Protease inhibitors such as Promogran consist of oxidised regenerated cellulose and collagen. They inhibit proteases in the wound and protect endogenous growth factors. In a 12 week study of 184 patients, 37% of Promogran treated patients healed compared with 28% of saline gauze treated patients, a non-significant difference.

Hyaluronic acid ester (Hyaff) is a fibrous ester of hyaluronic acid, which is a polysaccharide that is integral to the extracellular matrix and controls hydration and osmo-regulation. When Hyaff is applied to the wound, hyaluronic acid is released. It is useful in treating neuropathic ulcers complicated by sinuses.

Special wounds

DECUBITUS WOUNDS INCLUDING HEEL ULCERS

Heel ulcers can be off-loaded by foam wedges or pressure relief ankle foot orthoses (PRAFO).

The PRAFO (Fig. 4.23) is a ready-made orthotic device which has washable fleece liner with an aluminium and polypropylene

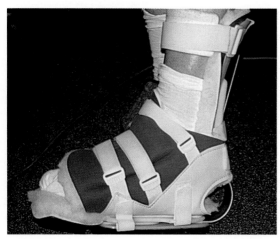

Fig. 4.23
The pressure relief ankle foot orthosis (PRAFO) relieves pressure on the back of the heel.

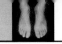

adjustable frame and a non-slip walking neoprene base. It is used to relieve pressure over the posterior aspect of the heel and maintain the ankle joint in a suitable position, thus preventing decubitus ulceration, aiding healing and preventing deformity. The patient can walk a little in the PRAFO.

Regular turning and repositioning of immobile patients to relieve continuous local ischaemia over pressure points is crucial in the prevention and management of diabetic heel ulcers. Special pressure-relieving mattresses are also useful.

BULLAE

Bullae are superficial fluid-filled sacs which develop when the skin is traumatised. There is controversy over the procedure of de-roofing bullae. Our practice is to drain tense bullae and all bullae more than one centimetre in diameter (Figs. 4.24a and b).

PUNCTURE WOUND

These are penetrating wounds, usually caused by sharp objects which may break off in the wound. The foot should be X-rayed but some objects, such as splinters of wood, are not radio-opaque. Ultrasound examination may then be useful. Any foreign body should be removed. Close follow up is required and prophylactic antibiotics are advised.

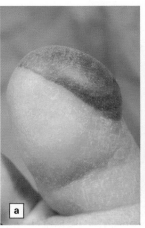 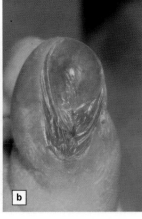

Fig. 4.24
(a) Tense bulla on hallux
(b) Bulla drained and decompressed by the podaitrist with a scalpel.

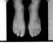

BURNS

Partial-thickness burns are allowed to heal by secondary intention as are some full-thickness burns. Extensive wounds need skin grafting. These are very susceptible to infection and antibiotics are prescribed as for ulcers (see below). Full-thickness burns should be referred to specialist burns centres.

ARTIFACTUAL WOUND

This is a difficult condition to treat and involvement of a psychiatrist with a special interest in artifactual disorders may be useful. Patients are aware of what they are doing but have little insight into their motives. They injure themselves with impunity because of neuropathy. Tamper-free dressings or casts which cannot be removed by the patient may provide the best opportunity for short-term healing, but the long-term outlook is bleak. Confrontation and admonishment are unhelpful as patients will just go elsewhere for their care.

Microbiological control

Now that the skin is broken, the Stage 3 patient is at great risk of infection as there is a clear portal of entry for invading bacteria. In the presence of neuropathy and ischaemia the inflammatory response is impaired. The patient lacks protective pain sensation which would otherwise automatically force him to rest. This state of affairs is a recipe for disaster unless effective microbiological surveillance is carried out.

We use the following plan for neuropathic and neuroischaemic ulcers based on many years of clinical experience and significant amputation reductions.

- As clinical signs of infection can be greatly diminished in the diabetic foot, close attention is paid to the results of ulcer swabs, which are taken at the first visit and at each subsequent visit, after debridement. Ulcer swabs give an indication of the type of bacteria that are present, which may progress from colonization to active infection. Antibiotics are prescribed more readily for the neuroischaemic foot as we have seen untreated infection often lead rapidly to necrosis and major amputation in this type of foot

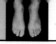

- Neuropathic ulcer: at the first visit, if the base of the ulcer is clean and a healthy pink colour, and there is no cellulitis, discharge or sinus present, then debridement, cleaning with saline, application of dressing and daily inspections will suffice
- Neuroischaemic ulcer: at the first visit, if the ulcer is superficial, oral amoxicillin 500 mg t.d.s. and flucloxacillin 500 mg q.d.s. to cover Gram-positive organisms are prescribed. (If the patient is penicillin allergic, prescribe clarithromycin 500 mg b.d. or cephadroxyl 1 g b.d. Clarithromycin may increase serum levels of statins, leading to myopathy and it is best to avoid it if the patient is taking statins). If the ulcer extends to the subcutaneous tissue, then trimethoprim 200 mg b.d. or ciprofloxacin 500 mg b.d. to cover gram negatives and metronidazole 400 mg t.d.s. to cover anaerobes are added to the above therapy
- The patient is reviewed within 1 week, together with the result of the ulcer swab
- If the neuropathic ulcer is healing well, treatment is continued without antibiotics
- If either the neuropathic or neuroischaemic ulcer has not improved and the swab is positive, the patient is treated with the appropriate antibiotic according to antibiotic sensitivities. In some cases of severe ischaemia, antibiotics are continued until the ulcer is healed.

It is important to maintain close clinical and microbiological surveillance of the ulcer to detect infection. At every patient visit, examination for local signs of infection, cellulitis or osteomyelitis is performed. If these are found, action is taken as described in Chapter 5. Early treatment is particularly important in the neuroischaemic foot to prevent infection leading to overwhelming necrosis.

Vascular control

If ulcers in the neuroischaemic foot fail to heal despite optimum treatment, the reason may be ischaemia. A careful vascular assessment is necessary to assess the degree of ischaemia, and to decide when to perform invasive investigations with a view to revascularization.

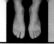

Initially the ankle brachial pressure index should be measured, supplemented by assessment of the Doppler waveform. Further tests such as measurement of transcutaneous oxygen tension and toe pressure may be helpful.

Pressure index

We accept that there is criticism of the pressure index. If arteries are calcified, it may be artifactually raised but we still feel that it is very relevant to the investigation of the diabetic foot as long as one understands the difficulties of its interpretation.

Thus, if the pressure index is 0.5, then it is low, and indicates severe ischaemia, whether the foot arteries are calcified or not. Indeed, if it is calcified, the true pressure index may be lower and even more urgent action is required.

Difficulty comes at pressure indices of 0.5 and above. However, one should always pay attention to the Doppler waveform, either in audible or visible form. The normal waveform is pulsatile (Fig. 4.25a) with a positive forward flow in systole followed by a short reverse flow and a further forward flow in diastole, but in the presence of arterial narrowing the waveform shows a reduced forward flow and is described as damped (Fig. 4.25b).

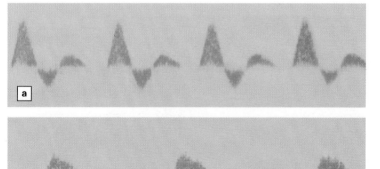

Fig. 4.25
(a) Doppler waveform from normal foot showing normal triphasic pattern.
(b) Doppler waveform from neuroischaemic foot showing damped pattern.

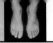

Transcutaneous oxygen tension

This measurement is a non-invasive method for monitoring arterial oxygen tension and reflects local arterial perfusion pressure. It is measured on the dorsum of the foot. A reading below 30 mmHg indicates severe ischaemia and the need for revascularization but levels can be falsely lowered by oedema and cellulitis (Fig. 4.26).

Toe pressure

Toe pressure can also be measured and a value below 30 mmHg indicates severe ischaemia.

Vascular Intervention

ANGIOGRAPHY AND ANGIOPLASTY

If an ischaemic ulcer has not shown progress in healing despite optimum treatment and:

- Ankle brachial pressure index is less than 0.5 or the Doppler waveform is damped
- Transcutaneous oxygen is less than 30 mmHg
- Toe pressure is less than 30 mmHg;

then angiography should ideally be carried out promptly. The decision to proceed to angiography is made in the joint Vascular

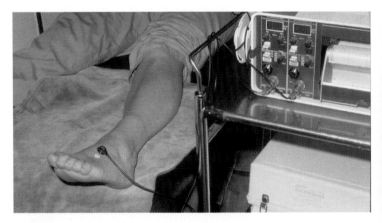

Fig. 4.26
Measurement of transcutaneous oxygen tension over dorsum of foot.

clinic and is performed by a duplex examination, which combines the features of Doppler waveform analysis with ultrasound imaging to produce a picture of arterial flow dynamics and morphology (Fig. 4.27). The duplex angiogram will show sites of arterial disease from the iliac arteries downwards. This information will determine whether intervention is required and also the mode of intervention. In most cases, arterial disease will be below the inguinal ligament and then an antegrade downstream femoral angiogram with digital subtraction imaging can be performed. This can be immediately followed by angioplasty of stenoses as well as occlusions throughout the femoral, popliteal and tibial vessels to achieve straight line arterial flow to the foot. In the rare cases of iliac disease, further imaging may be necessary either by retrograde femoral angiography or by magnetic resonance angiography (MRA). The advantages of MRA against conventional angiography are that there is no need for an

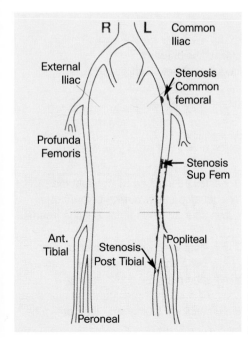

Fig. 4.27
Print-out of Duplex examination showing stenoses in the left common femoral artery, superficial femoral artery and posterior tibial artery.

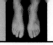

intra-arterial catheter and nephrotoxic contrast can be avoided. Thus, with suitable iliac imaging available, upstream angioplasty with possible iliac stenting may be performed.

Angioplasty is tolerated well and can be carried out in very elderly patients. In the event of re-stenosis, angioplasty is easily repeatable to achieve straight line flow to the foot. In suitable patients it is now possible to carry out transfemoral angiography and angioplasty as an outpatient procedure. A small bore needle is used, and after the procedure the puncture site is closed by a special 'Perclose' technique which is a suture mediated closure of the arterial access site. This allows the patient to sit up after two hours and to walk in four hours.

Contraindications to day case angiography include:

- Myocardial infarction/cerebrovascular event within last six months
- Severe cardiac/respiratory disease
- Major surgery within last month
- Warfarin therapy
- Renal failure.

PREPARATIONS FOR TRANSFEMORAL ANGIOGRAPHY

Angiography is a safe procedure with few complications.
Pre-procedure Investigations should include:

- Full blood count, including a platelet count
- Blood coagulation indices
- Serum electrolytes and creatinine
- Blood grouping.

Metformin may aggravate renal failure induced by contrast media. Patients taking metformin should stop this two days before the procedure and restart two days after, or when renal function returns to normal.

It is important to keep the patient well hydrated. Patients with chronic renal insufficiency have been shown to be protected against contrast media-induced renal nephropathy by administering acetylcysteine. All patients should have their renal function assessed prior to angioplasty. If serum creatinine >120mmol/L, then prescribe

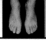

acetylcysteine 600 mg orally bd for one day pre-procedure and up to two days post-procedure (usual 48 hour total duration). Ideally the first dose should be 12 hours pre-procedure. Concurrent hydration is essential in these patients. Renal function should be re-checked 24 hours post procedure. We no longer use pre- and peri-operative dopamine.

Blood coagulation indices should also be checked. If the patient has previously been on warfarin then this must be stopped at least three days prior to the procedure and the patient changed to intravenous heparin. The heparin infusion is stopped two hours before the procedure.

Insulin-dependent patients are placed first on the list in outpatient angiography and have their insulin after the procedure is finished.

ARTERIAL BYPASS

If lesions are too widespread for angioplasty, then arterial bypass may be considered. However, this is a major, sometimes lengthy, operation not without risk, and is more commonly reserved to treat severe tissue infection and destruction which cannot be managed without the restoration of pulsatile blood flow to the foot (see Chapter 6).

PAIN RELIEF

In general, the neuroischaemic foot is not painful; however, in a few cases when neuropathy is mild the patient suffers pain from the ulcer as well as rest pain, particularly at night. It is important to control this and advice should be sought from the Pain Team.

- An opioid such as dihydrocodeine, alone (30 mg every 4-6 hours) or in combination with a non-opioid analgesic, co-dydramol (dihydrocodeine 10 mg, paracetamol 500 mg, two tablets every 4–6 hours) may be useful in moderate pain
- Tramadol (50–100 mg 4-6 hourly) is an opioid derivative, which is often less sedating and less constipating than codeine
- Tricyclic antidepressants, for example dothiepin 50–100 mg at night, are useful at relieving rest pain in bed.

When pain is severe, it is important to give regular morphine therapy.

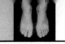

The initial dose of modified release preparations, devised for twice-daily administration is 10–20 mg every 12 hours, if no other analgesic or paracetamol has been previously prescribed. However, if it is replacing a weaker opioid analgesic, for example co-dydramol, the initial dose should be 20–30 mg every 12 hours. The doses should be gradually increased but the frequency kept at every 12 hours. If breakthrough pain occurs between the 12-hourly doses, then morphine, as oral solution (Oramorph 5–20 mg every 4 hours) or standard formulation tablets such as Sevredol 10–50 mg every 4 hours, can be given. An opioid derivative, oxycodone, can be useful in relieving moderate to severe pain. A new approach is to use skin patches containing opioids which are delivered transdermally and can last from 48 to 72 hours.

- When using any opioid-like drugs, beware of respiratory depression, to which diabetic patients with autonomic neuropathy can be susceptible
- We try to avoid non-steroid anti-inflammatory drugs and cyclo-oxygenase-2 inhibitors as they may cause renal impairment and worsen cardiac function leading to congestive heart failure
- Chemical sympathectomy by paravertebral injection of phenol is also used to relieve rest pain although it does not increase peripheral blood flow
- If patients do come to major amputation, then a lumbar epidural block with bupivicaine should be started 48 hours beforehand to relieve perioperative pain.

Metabolic control

It is important to make sure that there is no systemic, metabolic or nutritional disturbance to retard healing of the ulcer.

The patient needs the following:

- Full blood count to exclude anaemia
- Serum electrolytes and serum creatinine, to assess renal function
- Liver function tests to obtain baseline of liver enzymes before starting possible antibiotic therapy and to measure serum albumin as an indicator of nutrition (< 3.5 g/L indicates malnutrition and dietary advice should be obtained)

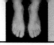

- Wound healing and neutrophil function is impaired by hyperglycaemia, which should be controlled as tightly as possible. Type 2 patients on oral hypoglycaemic therapy with sub-optimal control which cannot be corrected should be started on insulin
- Hyperlipidaemia, hypertension and smoking should be actively treated. Patients with neuroischaemic ulcers should be on statin therapy as well as antiplatelet therapy. Diabetic patients who are above 55 years and have peripheral vascular disease should also benefit from an angiotensin-converting enzyme (ACE) inhibitor to prevent further vascular episodes
- When managing hypertension in the presence of leg ischaemia, it is important to achieve a fine balance between maintaining a pressure that improves perfusion of the ischaemic limb while reducing the blood pressure enough to limit the risk of cardiovascular complications. However, beta-blockers, such as bisoprolol, have been shown to increase survival in cardiac failure and are not contraindicated in patients with neuroischaemic feet
- Many patients with diabetic foot problems will have evidence of cardiac failure. Aggressive treatment with angiotensin-converting enzyme inhibitors, diuretics, beta-blockers and aldosterone antagonists will improve tissue perfusion and also reduce swelling of the feet
- Renal impairment may also be present, and optimum treatment is essential to control lower limb swelling.

Educational control

Patients who lack protective pain sensation need to know that foot ulcers are a important problem but that they will heal with optimal care. The following educational material – aimed directly at patients – seeks to clarify common misconceptions about ulcers and their management. It is important to judge how much information the patient can take on board to allow maximum co-operation between patient and the diabetic foot team. This is difficult in patients with psychiatric disease and cognitive disabilities when the approach must be specifically tailored to the patient.

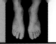

Patient information

FOOT ULCERS

- Foot ulcers can be a very serious problem. It is essential to heal them quickly
- Nerve damage from diabetes can reduce pain: therefore, a foot ulcer may not be painful, so it is easy to ignore. Most serious health problems are painful or make patients feel ill. By the time a foot ulcer hurts or gives symptoms of illness it has seriously damaged your foot
- To give your ulcer the best chance of healing quickly, please follow this advice.

REST

- When you walk, every step is like hitting your ulcer with a hammer. It helps to use crutches, a Zimmer or a wheelchair to take the weight right off your ulcer
- Special shoes and insoles, plaster casts or removable braces can take the load off your foot if it is essential for you to walk a little.

TREATING YOUR ULCER

- Ulcers gather debris and dead tissue around them, and some develop hard skin
- Unless ulcers are cleaned by cutting away all the debris and hard skin, they can become choked and they will not heal quickly
- It can be helpful to clean up the edges until they bleed a little. This gives the ulcer a fresh start. You should never try to do this for yourself: it is the job of the doctor or podiatrist.

DRESSINGS

- Keep your ulcer covered by a dressing to keep it clean and warm
- It will need a quick check every day to be sure it is healing well and not infected

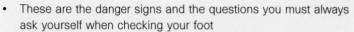

- These are the danger signs and the questions you must always ask yourself when checking your foot
  (a) Swelling – has your shoe become tight?
  (b) Colour change – is there redness of the skin around the ulcer? Are there bluish marks like bruises or is the skin going black?
  (c) Has the ulcer itself changed colour?
  (d) Discharge – has your ulcer become wet where it was dry before? Is there blood or pus discharging from it?
  (e) Have you developed any new ulcers or blistering?
  (f) Has your ulcer become painful or uncomfortable or is your foot throbbing?
  (g) Do you feel unwell with fever, flu-like symptoms or poorly controlled diabetes?
- If the answer to any question is yes, then the foot should be checked the same day either by your doctor or the diabetic foot clinic
- If you cannot reach your feet or see them clearly, ask your family or a friend to help you with checking and dressing your foot ulcer, or your doctor can ask a nurse to help you.

Chapter 5

Managing Stage 4: the infected foot

PRESENTATION AND DIAGNOSIS

The diabetic patient enters Stage 4 because the foot is now infected and microbiological control has been lost. At no other stage in the natural history of the diabetic foot is early diagnosis and intervention so important. Twenty four hours of undiagnosed and untreated infection can destroy the diabetic foot.

The most common manifestation is cellulitis, defined as an infection of skin and subcutaneous tissue, usually secondary to an ulcer, and presenting as redness or erythema. However, Stage 4 covers a spectrum of presentations under the general heading of infection. These range from local infection of the ulcer through to sloughing of soft tissue and vascular compromise of the skin, seen as a blue discolouration, secondary to reduced blood supply to the skin. This spectrum occurs in both neuropathic and neuroischaemic feet but in the presence of neuropathy and ischaemia signs of inflammation are often diminished. There is a reduced host response to infection which is particularly noticeable in diabetic patients with impaired renal and liver function.

There are two crucial decisions to be made when managing infected diabetic feet: first, to decide on the presence of infection so as to start antibiotic therapy rapidly, and secondly, to decide whether the patient needs surgical debridement to remove extensive infected tissue. Often the latter is a very difficult decision. It should be clearly understood that diabetic feet can be severely infected and need operative removal of infected tissue yet may not exhibit the classical signs of fluctuance and abscess formation. All patients presenting with clinical signs of infection should have an X-ray of the foot to detect:

- Gas in the deep tissues
- Foreign body
- Bony destruction, secondary to infection
- Charcot osteoarthropathy.

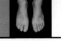

For descriptive purposes the infected diabetic foot can be divided into the locally infected ulcer, mild infection and severe infection. Any of these presentations may be complicated by osteomyelitis.

Locally infected ulcer

Local signs that an ulcer has become infected include:

- The base of the ulcer changes from healthy pink granulations to yellowish or grey tissue and becomes moist (Fig. 5.1)
- Purulent discharge
- Unpleasant smell
- Sinuses develop in an ulcer
- Edges may become undermined
- Bone or tendon becomes exposed.

Mild infection

- This presents as erythema, warmth and swelling usually associated with ulceration (Fig. 5.2)
- In the pigmented (e.g. Afro-Caribbean) foot, cellulitis can be difficult to detect, but careful comparison with the other foot may reveal a tawny hue
- In the neuroischaemic foot, it may be difficult to differentiate between the erythema of cellulitis and the redness of ischaemia. However, the redness of ischaemia is usually cold, although not always so and is most marked on dependency, while the erythema of inflammation is warm
- Erythematous inflammation of the feet also occurs in eczema, which is characterised by crusting and scaling. This is not seen in cellulitis
- Erythema also occurs in response to traumas, including insect stings.

Severe infection

- There is an intense widespread erythema and swelling. Lymphangitis (Fig 5.3), regional lymphadenitis, malaise, flu-like symptoms, fever and rigors may be present

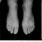

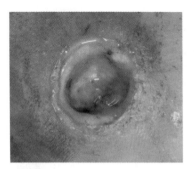

Fig. 5.1
Local infection: the base of the ulcer
has changed from pink to grey.

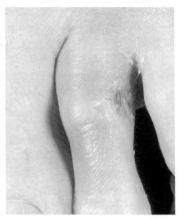

Fig. 5.2
Mild cellulitis around ulcer.

- In the presence of neuropathy, pain and throbbing are often absent, but if present, usually indicate pus within the tissues. Palpation may reveal fluctuance, suggesting abscess formation, but discrete abscesses are relatively uncommon in the infected diabetic foot

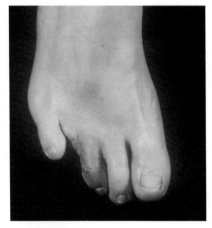

Fig. 5.3
Lymphangitis spreading from the
3rd toe. The 4th toe has been
amputated.

Many inexperienced surgeons are unaware of this and feel that the only indication for operation is fluctuance with abscess formation. This is rare in the diabetic foot because the poor white cell function cannot localize the infection to create an abscess

- Often there is a generalized sloughing of the ulcer and surrounding subcutaneous tissues which eventually liquefy and disintegrate
- Puncture wounds may be complicated by cellulitis. Bacteria are inoculated at the base of the puncture wound and then track back towards the surface of the skin, with infection eventually manifesting itself as a cellulitis
- Infection can also present as a blue–purple discolouration when there is an inadequate supply of oxygen to the soft tissues. This is caused by increased metabolic demands of infection and a reduction of blood flow to the skin
- Blue discolouration can occur in both the neuropathic and also the neuroischaemic foot, particularly in the toes (Figs 5.4a and b) and in the neuroischaemic foot must not be automatically attributed to worsening ischaemia
- In very severe cases of infection, bluish–purplish discolouration of the skin indicates subcutaneous necrosis (Fig. 5.5). Severe subcutaneous infection by Gram-negative and anaerobic organisms produces gas, which can be detected by palpating crepitus and can be seen on X-ray (Fig. 5.6)
- Only 50% of episodes of severe infections will provoke a fever or leucocytosis. However serum C-reactive protein is a good indicator of the extent of infection and a subsequent fall in its level during treatment is a useful monitor of resolution of infection.

These three presentations may be complicated by underlying osteomyelitis.

Osteomyelitis
- Osteomyelitis should be diagnosed by inserting a sterile probe into the ulcer. If it penetrates to bone, this confirms the diagnosis
- A sign that an underlying joint is involved is the drainage of viscous, bubbly synovial fluid which is clear and sometimes has a yellowish tinge

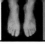

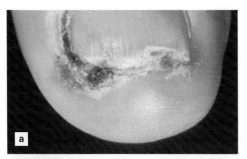

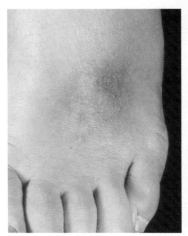

Fig. 5.4
(a) Blue discolouration in the first toe of neuroischaemic foot secondary to infection.
(b) Blue toe has become pink after treatment of infection with antibiotics.

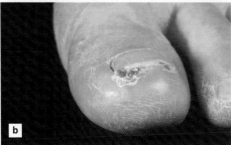

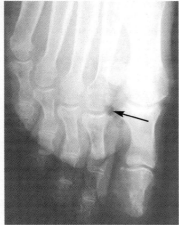

Fig. 5.5
Purplish discolouration indicating subcutaneous necrosis.

Fig. 5.6
Gas in the tissues (arrowed) in severe soft tissue infection.

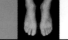

- Chronic osteomyelitis of a toe has a swollen, red, sausage-like appearance
- In the initial stages, plain X-ray may be normal. Signs of osteomyelitis such as localized loss of bone density or cortical outline (Fig. 5.7), may not be apparent for at least 14 days. MRI scanning may detect early changes (Figs. 5.8a and b).

MANAGEMENT

Infection in the diabetic foot needs full multidisciplinary treatment. It is vital to achieve:

- Microbiological control
- Wound control
- Vascular control

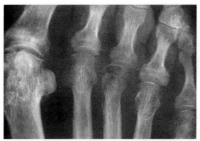

Fig. 5.7
Osteomyelitis in third metatarsal head with loss of bone density and cortical outline.

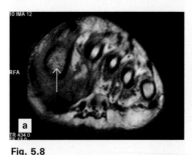
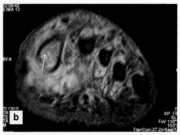

Fig. 5.8
Osteomyelitis in first metatarsal head. (a) T1 sequence shows reduced signal in the fatty marrow of the first metatarsal head (arrowed) compared with other metatarsal heads. (b) Increased uptake on STIR sequence in first metatarsal head (arrowed) indicating oedema. This is more pronounced compared with other metatarsal heads.

- Mechanical control
- Metabolic control
- Educational control.

If infection is not controlled, it can spread with alarming rapidity, and can cause extensive tissue necrosis, taking the foot into Stage 5 or Stage 6.

Microbiological control
General principles
The microbiology of the diabetic foot is unique. Infection can be caused by Gram-positive, Gram-negative and anaerobic bacteria, singly or in combination (Table 5.1).

Antibiotics alone do not always treat foot infections successfully. Severe infection in the diabetic foot may be accompanied by deep soft tissue involvement which spreads along the fascial planes and needs early extensive surgical debridement and concomitant antibiotic therapy. At initial presentation, it is important to prescribe a wide spectrum of antibiotics because it is impossible to predict the organisms from the clinical appearance. It is therefore vital to send

Bacteria isolated from the diabetic foot	
Gram-positive	**Gram-negative**
Staphylococcus aureus	Proteus
Streptococcus (often Group B)	Klebsiella
Enterococcus	Enterobacter
	Escherichia coli
Anaerobes	Pseudomonas aeruginosa
Bacteroides	Citrobacter
Clostridium	Morganella morganii
Peptostreptococcus	Serratia
Peptococcus	Acinetobacter

Table 5.1
Bacteria isolated from the diabetic foot.

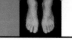

swabs for culture without delay in all Stage 4 patients. Deep swabs or tissue should be taken from the ulcer after initial debridement and if the patient undergoes operative debridement then deep tissue should also be sent. Ulcer swabs should be taken at every follow-up visit. Blood cultures should be sent if there is fever and systemic toxicity.

As there is a poor immune response of the diabetic patient to sepsis, even bacteria regarded as skin commensals may cause severe tissue damage. This includes Gram-negative organisms such as *Citrobacter*, *Serratia* and *Pseudomonas*. When Gram-negative bacteria are isolated from an ulcer swab they should not be regarded automatically as insignificant. Group A streptococcus is a rare isolate from ulcers but when present can cause severe systemic upset. Good communication with the microbiologist is advised. When a positive culture is found, it is necessary to focus antibiotic therapy according to sensitivities. Useful antibiotics are shown in Table 5.2.

Antibiotic treatment

Infection in the neuroischaemic foot is often more serious than in the neuropathic foot which has a good arterial blood supply; therefore we regard a positive ulcer swab in a neuroischaemic foot as having serious implications, and this influences antibiotic policy. Antibiotic treatment is discussed both as initial treatment and follow-up treatment and is divided into treatment of the infected ulcer and the foot with mild infection, and the foot with severe infection. We regard the infected ulcer and the foot with mild cellulitis as of equally serious import and have therefore grouped them together. There are different sections covering treatment of the neuropathic foot and treatment of the neuroischaemic foot. Treatment of osteomyelitis is also discussed. Diabetic patients with renal impairment are particularly susceptible to infection but their antibiotic dosages will need to be reduced in renal failure (Table 5.3).

We recommend the aggressive use of antibiotics in Stage 4, but keep a very close surveillance for side-effects, particularly vomiting and diarrhoea. If this does occur, it is advisable to stop the antibiotics, at least for a short period, to prevent the development of clostridium difficile colitis. Faeces should be sent for culture but therapy should be started immediately with either vancomycin 125mg q.d.s. orally (IV

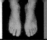

Useful antibiotics

Micro-organism	Antibiotic treatment	
	Oral	Intravenous
Streptococcus *(inc. Group B, C & G)*	Amoxicillin 500 mg t.d.s. Clarithromycin 500 mg b.d. Clindamycin 300 mg q.d.s.	Amoxicillin 500 mg t.d.s. Clindamycin 300 mg q.d.s.
Staphylococcus aureus	Flucloxacillin 500 mg q.d.s. Sodium fusidate 500 mg t.d.s. Clindamycin 300 mg q.d.s. Rifampicin 300 mg t.d.s.	Flucloxacillin 500 mg q.d.s. Gentamicin 5 mg/kg/day *(according to levels)* Clindamycin 300 mg q.d.s.
Anaerobes	Metronidazole 400 mg t.d.s. Clindamycin 300 mg q.d.s.	Metronidazole 500 mg t.d.s. Clindamycin 300 mg q.d.s.
Gram negatives	Ciprofloxacin 500 mg b.d. Cefadroxil 1 g b.d. Trimethoprim 200 mg b.d.	Ceftazidime 1–2 g t.d.s. Ceftriaxone 1–2 g daily Gentamicin 5 mg/kg/day *(according to levels)* Piperacillin–tazobactam 4.5 g t.d.s. Meropenem 500 mg t.d.s.
MRSA	Sodium fusidate 500 mg t.d.s. Trimethoprim 200 mg b.d. Rifampicin 300 mg t.d.s. Doxycycline 100 mg daily Linezolid 600 mg b.d.	Vancomycin 1 g b.d *(according to levels)* Teicoplanin 400 mg daily Linezolid 600 mg b.d.

Intramuscular antibiotics:
Ceftriaxone 1 g daily IM to treat Gram-positives and Gram-negatives
Teicoplanin 400 mg daily IM to treat Gram-positives including MRSA
Imipenem w. cilastatin 500 mg b.d. IM to treat Gram-positives, Gram-negatives and anaerobes

Table 5.2
Antibiotics for treating the infected foot, including intramuscular antibiotics that can be given at home.

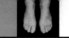

Table 5.3 Antibiotic dosage in renal failure

Antibiotic	Dose for normal renal function	Mild impairment (serum Cr 120 –200 µmol/L)	Moderate impairment (serum Cr 200–400 µmol/L)	Severe impairment (serum Cr>400 µmol/L)
Amikacin	iv 7.5 mg/kg/bd	Give 7.5mg/kg daily redose <5mg/L	Give 7.5 mg/kg daily redose <5mg/L	Give 7.5mg/kg daily redose < 5mg/L
Amoxicillin	iv/po 500mg tds	No change	No change	500mg bd
Benzylpenicillin	iv 1.2g qds	No change	75% of normal dose	Maximum 3.6g daily
Cefadroxil	po 0.5–1g bd	0.5–1g bd	0.5–1g daily	0.5–1g daily
Ceftazidime	iv 1–2g tds	1g 12 hrly	0.5–1g 24 hrly	0.5–1g 48 hrly
Ceftriaxone	iv 1–4g daily	No adjustment	No adjustment	1–2g daily
Cefuroxime	iv 750 mg to 1.5g tds	No adjustment	750mg to 1.5g bd	750mg bd
Ciprofloxacin	iv 100–400mg bd po 250–750mg bd	No adjustment po max 500mg bd	iv 100–200mgbd po max 500mg bd	iv 100–200mgbd po max 500mg bd
Clindamycin	iv 150–600mg qds po 150–450mg qds	No adjustment No adjustment	No adjustment No adjustment	No adjustment No adjustment
Clarithromycin	iv 500mg bd po 500mg bd	No adjustment	No adjustment	iv 250mg bd po 250mg bd
Doxycycline	po First day 200mg then 100 mg daily	No adjustment	No adjustment	No adjustment
Flucloxacillin	iv 500mg qds po 500mg qds	No adjustment No adjustment	No adjustment No adjustment	500mg td.s. 500mg td.s.
Gentamicin	iv 5 mg/kg once daily	1.5–2mg/kg redose <1mg/L	1.5–2mg/kg redose <1mg/L	1.5–2mg/kg redose <1mg/L
Meropenem	iv 500 mg to 1g tds	500 mg to 1g 12 hrly	250–500mg 12hrly	250–500mg 24 hrly
Metronidazole	iv 500mg tds po 400mg tds	No adjustment No adjustment	No adjustment No adjustment	No adjustment No adjustment
Rifampicin	po 600mg bd	No adjustment	No adjustment	No adjustment
Sodium fusidate	iv 500mg tds po 500mg tds	No adjustment No adjustment	No adjustment No adjustment	No adjustment No adjustment
Tazocin	iv 2.25–4.5g tds	2.25–4.5g tds	2.25–4.5 g bd	2.25–4.5 g bd
Teicoplanin	iv load with 400mg 12 hrly iv then 400 mg daily	Load first then 200mg once daily	Load first then 200 mg alt. days	Load first then 200 mg 3x/week
Trimethoprim	po 100–200mg bd	200mg bd then half dose	normal for 3 days then half dose	Half normal dose
Vancomycin	iv 1 g bd trough < 10mg/L	Give 1g: redose when level <10mg/L	Give 1g: redose when level < 10mg/L	Give 1g: redose when level < 10mg/L

Antibiotic	HD	CAPD	CAVH
Amikacin	Give 7.5mg/kg daily redose <5mg/L	Give 7.5mg/kg daily redose < 5mg/L	Give 7.5mg/kg daily redose <5 mg/L
Amoxicillin	500 mg bd	500 mg bd	500 mg tds
Benzylpenicillin	Maximum 3.6g daily	Maximum 3.6g daily	50% of normal dose
Cefadroxil	0.5–1 g daily	0.5–1g daily	Not applicable
Ceftazidime	0.5–1 g 48 hrly	0.5–1g 48 hrly	1–2 g daily
Ceftriaxone	1–2 g daily	1–2g daily	1–2 g daily
Cefuroxime	750mg bd	750 mg bd	750 mg bd
Ciprofloxacin	iv 100–200mg bd po max 500mg bd	iv 100–200mgbd po max 500mg bd	iv 200 mg bd po max 500 mg bd
Clarithromycin	iv 250mg bd po 250mg bd	iv 250mg bd po 250 mg bd	iv 250mg bd po 250mg bd

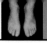

Table 5.3 (continued)

Antibiotic	HD	CAPD	CAVH
Clindamycin	No adjustment	No adjustment	No adjustment
Doxycycline	No adjustment	No adjustment	No adjustment
Flucloxacillin	500 mg tds	500 mg tds	500 mg qds
Gentamicin	1.5–2 mg/kg redose < 1 mg/L	1.5–2 mg/kg redose < 1 mg/L	1.5–2 mg/kg redose < 1 mg/L
Meropenem	250–500 mg 24 hrly	250–500 mg 24 hrly	250–500 mg 12 hrly
Metronidazole	No adjustment	No adjustment	No adjustment
Rifampicin	No adjustment	No adjustment	No adjustment
Sodium fusidate	No adjustment	No adjustment	No adjustment
Tazocin	2.25–4.5 g bd	2.25–4.5 g bd	2.25–4.5 g tds
Teicoplanin	Load first then 200 mg 3 x/week	Load first then 200 mg 3 x/week	Load first then 200 mg alt. days
Trimethoprim	Half normal dose	Half normal dose	Half normal dose
Vancomycin	Give 1 g: redose when level < 10 mg/L	Give 1 g: redose when level < 10 mg/L	Give 1 g: redose when level < 10 mg/L

HD, haemodialysis; CAPD, continuous ambulatory peritoneal dialysis; CAVH, continuous arteriovenous haemofiltration; Cr, creatinine.

Table 5.3
Antibiotic dosage in renal failure (HD, haemodialysis; CAPD, continuous ambulatory peritoneal dialysis; CAVH, continuous arteriovenous haemofiltration; Cr, creatinine.).

vancomycin does not treat clostridium difficile) or metronidazole 400 mg td.s. orally. Acidophilus lactobacillus tablets can also be given to help to restore the intestinal bacterial flora. We advise our patients to eat live yoghurt when taking antibiotics. In severe cases of clostridium difficile infection, there is abdominal pain associated with diarrhoea and often a raised white blood cell count and fever. Patients may need hospitalization and intravenous fluids. A useful diagnostic investigation is an abdominal CT scan which will reveal loops of oedematous large bowel.

When patients with foot infections develop diarrhoea with a high white blood cell count and fever, it is a difficult to know whether the fever and raised white cell count are due to either worsening of the foot infection or the onset of clostridium difficile diarrhoea. Close examination of the foot will determine whether infection here has worsened. If this is not the case, then the high white cell count and fever are likely to be due to colitis and the antibiotics should be stopped immediately.

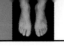

Another cause of a high white cell count and fever in a diabetic patient taking antibiotics is candidal infection including candidal septicaemia. Diabetic patients with indwelling tunnelled lines, such as Hickmann lines, are particularly susceptible to this complication, which will need active treatment with anti-fungal agents such as fluconazole. Indeed, in diabetic foot patients, tunnelled lines may also be associated with metastatic infections, including discitis. For this reason, we try to avoid them in our patients, and we have used intramuscular injections of antibiotics in the community. In the hospital, PICC (peripherally inserted central catheter) lines are increasingly used in patients with 'difficult' veins and are left in situ for two or three weeks.

LOCAL ULCER INFECTION AND MILD INFECTION IN THE NEUROPATHIC FOOT

INITIAL TREATMENT

These patients are suitable for outpatient care and oral antibiotics.

- Give amoxicillin 500 mg t.d.s., flucloxacillin 500 mg q.d.s., metronidazole 400 mg t.d.s. and ciprofloxacin 500 mg b.d. If the patient is allergic to penicillin, substitute clarithromycin 500 mg b.d. for amoxicillin and flucloxacillin
- Infection on the borderline of mild to severe, can be treated with ceftriaxone 1 g in 3.5 mL 1% lidocaine IM daily. This route of antibiotics is also useful when oral antibiotics have not been efficacious. It should not be used for those patients taking anticoagulants.

FOLLOW-UP PLAN (Table 5.4)

- If no signs of infection and no organisms isolated, stop antibiotics
- If no signs of infection are present but organisms are isolated, focus antibiotics, and review in one week
- If signs of infection are present but no organisms are isolated, continue the antibiotics as above
- If signs of infection are still present, and organisms are isolated, focus antibiotics according to sensitivities
- If methicillin-resistant *Staphylococcus aureus* (MRSA) is grown, but there are no local or systemic signs of infection, use topical mupirocin 2% ointment (if sensitive)

Follow-up plan – neuropathic foot		
Signs of infection	**Organisms**	**Antibiotics**
No	No	Stop
No	Yes	Focus
Yes	No	Continue
Yes	Yes	Focus
No	MRSA	Topical
Yes	MRSA	Focus

Table 5.4
Follow-up plan – neuropathic foot.

- If MRSA is grown with local signs of infection, consider oral therapy with two of the following: sodium fusidate 500 mg t.d.s., rifampicin 300 mg t.d.s., trimethoprim 200 mg b.d. and doxycycline 100mg daily according to sensitivities, with topical mupirocin 2% ointment. Linezolid is a new antibiotic with good activity against Gram-positive organisms including MRSA.

LOCAL SIGNS OF INFECTION IN THE ULCER AND MILD INFECTION IN THE NEUROISCHAEMIC FOOT

INITIAL TREATMENT
Suitable for outpatient care, but if patient is elderly, frail and lives alone arrange daily visit from a community nurse. Prescribe amoxicillin 500mg t.d.s., flucloxacillin 500 mg q.d.s., metronidazole 400 mg t.d.s. and ciprofloxacin 500 mg b.d. Infection on the borderline of mild to severe can be treated with ceftriaxone 1 g in 3.5 mL 1% lidocaine IM.

FOLLOW-UP PLAN (Table 5.5)
- If no signs of infection and no organisms grown, consider stopping antibiotics. However, if severely ischaemic and pressure index <0.5 and there is no possibility of revascularization, consider continuing antibiotics until healing (see Chapter 4)
- If no signs of infection, but organisms present, focus the antibiotics according to sensitivities

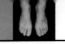

- If signs of infection present but no organisms grown, continue to give broad-spectrum antibiotics, with amoxicillin 500 mg t.d.s., flucloxacillin 500 mg q.d.s., metronidazole 400 mg t.d.s. and ciprofloxacin 500 mg b.d.
- If signs of infection are still present, and organisms are grown, focus the antibiotics according to sensitivities
- If MRSA is grown, whether signs of infection or not, consider oral therapy with two of the following: sodium fusidate 500 mg t.d.s., rifampicin 300 mg t.d.s., trimethoprim 200 mg b.d. and doxycycline 100 mg daily and topical therapy with mupirocin 2% ointment.

SEVERE INFECTION IN THE NEUROPATHIC AND NEUROISCHAEMIC FOOT

INITIAL TREATMENT

- Admission for intravenous antibiotics is the treatment of choice for this serious condition
- Quadruple therapy is indicated: amoxicillin 500 mg t.d.s. IV, flucloxacillin 500 mg q.d.s. IV, metronidazole 500 mg t.d.s. IV and ceftazidime 1 g t.d.s IV. If the patient shows systemic signs of infection, then one dose of gentamicin should be considered at 5 mg/Kg although this dosage should be reduced appropriately in renal failure
- If patient is allergic to penicillin, replace amoxicillin and flucloxacillin with clarithromycin 500 mg b.d. IV or vancomycin 1 g b.d. IV (with doses adjusted according to serum levels)
- On admission the foot should be urgently assessed as to the need for surgical debridement (see Wound control)
- If admission is not possible, then give ceftriaxone 1 g in 3.5 mL 1% lidocaine IM daily and metronidazole 400 mg t.d.s. orally. Trace the distribution of the cellulitis with a marker pen so that extension can be detected and review in two days
- Patients should be on bedrest at home with daily visits from a community nurse to redress the foot and alert the diabetic foot clinic if the foot is deteriorating
- On review as an outpatient, if cellulitis is controlled, continue ceftriaxone 1 g in 3.5 mL 1% lidocaine IM and metronidazole 400 mg t.d.s. orally, and review one week later.

Follow-up plan – neuroischaemic foot

Signs of infection	Organisms	Antibiotics
No	No	Stop*
No	Yes	Focus
Yes	No	Continue
Yes	Yes	Focus
No	MRSA	Focus
Yes	MRSA	Focus

Table 5.5
Follow-up plan – neuroischaemic foot. * If patient is severely ischaemic, continue antibiotics (see text).

FOLLOW-UP PLAN

- The infected foot should be inspected daily to gauge the initial response to antibiotic therapy
- Appropriate antibiotics should be selected when sensitivities are available
- If no organisms are isolated, and yet the foot remains severely cellulitic, then a repeat deep swab or tissue should be taken, but the quadruple antibiotic therapy, as above, should be continued
- If MRSA is isolated, give vancomycin 1 g b.d. IV, dosage to be adjusted according to serum levels, or teicoplanin 400 mg 12-hourly IV for three doses and then 400 mg daily. These antibiotics may need to be accompanied by either sodium fusidate 500 mg t.d.s. or rifampicin 300 mg t.d.s. orally
- Intravenous antibiotic therapy can be changed to the appropriate oral therapy when the signs of cellulitis have resolved
- Patients should be followed up weekly in the diabetic foot clinic and antibiotic therapy adjusted as described above.

OSTEOMYELITIS

INITIAL TREATMENT

- At first, antibiotics will be given for the infected foot as above
- On review, antibiotic selection is guided by the results of deep swabs or tissue, but it is useful to choose antibiotics with good bone penetration, such as sodium fusidate 500 mg t.d.s., rifampicin 300 mg t.d.s., clindamycin 300 mg q.d.s. and ciprofloxacin 500 mg b.d.

- Antibiotics should be given for at least 12 weeks. During this time, the ulcer will have regular debridement and bone fragments at the base of ulcer can be easily removed
- Such conservative therapy is often successful, and is associated with resolution of cellulitis and healing of the ulcer
- However, if after three months' treatment the ulcer persists, with continued probing to bone which is fragmented on X-ray, we favour resection of the underlying bone, which may entail toe amputation or removal of the metatarsal head.

Wound control
The neuropathic foot

Diabetic foot infections are almost always more extensive than would appear from initial examination and surface appearance. It is wise to perform an initial debridement in the diabetic foot clinic so that the true dimensions of the lesion can be revealed and tissue samples obtained for culture. Often callus may be overlying the ulcer and this must be removed to reveal the extent of the underlying ulcer and allow drainage of pus and removal of infected sloughy tissue (Figs. 5.9a,b,c,d). Infection should respond to intravenous antibiotics, but the patient needs daily review to detect evidence of spread. An outline of any area of cellulitis may be drawn on the foot so that extension of the cellulitic area can be detected quickly.

In severe episodes of infection, the ulcer may be complicated by extensive infected subcutaneous soft tissue. At this point, the tissue is not frankly necrotic but has started to break down and liquefy. It is best for this tissue to be removed operatively (Fig. 5.10). The definite indications for urgent surgical intervention are:

- Large area of infected sloughy tissue (Figs. 5.11a and b)
- Localized fluctuance and expression of pus (Figs. 5.12a and b)
- Crepitus with gas in the soft tissues on X-ray. However, gas immediately adjacent to an ulcer may have entered the foot through the ulcer and is of less importance than gas in the deep tissues of the foot or leg

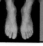

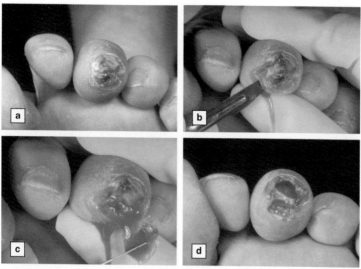

Fig. 5.9
Debridement in the foot clinic. (a) Cellulitic toe with apical callus. (b) Sharp debridement to remove callus. (c) Pus is drained. (d) The true dimensions of the lesion, which probed to bone, are exposed.

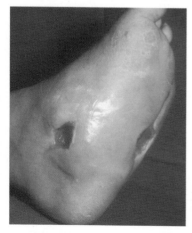

Fig. 5.10
Charcot foot with rocker-bottom ulcer debrided on medial and plantar aspects.

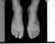

- Purplish discolouration of the skin, indicating subcutaneous necrosis (Figs. 5.13a,b,c).

There are two other indications for surgery in the management of the neuropathic foot namely osteomyelitis that has not responded to

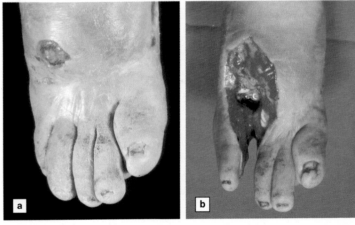

Fig. 5.11
(a) Severe cellulitis associated with deep infection. (b) Same foot after surgery to remove infected tissue.

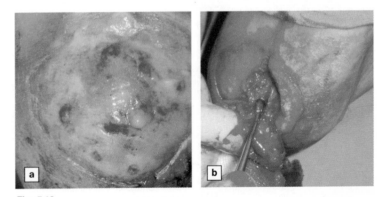

Fig. 5.12
(a) Pus exuding from plantar surface of cellulitic ulcerated heel. (b) Operative debridement with excision of infected tissue.

conservative measures and the development of collections of fluid or pus that are difficult to detect clinically. Magnetic resonance imaging (MRI) may be useful to look for the presence of osteomyelitis and also to detect collections of fluid (Figs. 5.14a,b,c). Intravenous injection of gadolinium-containing contrast agent heightens the sensitivity of the diagnosis of these clinical features as gadolinium concentrates in areas of inflammation. However, MRI has limitations and can show a number of false positive diagnoses.

The neuroischaemic foot

In severe infections, surgical debridement may also be necessary and similar criteria as for the neuropathic foot are used in the decision to operate. Any surgical debridement needs to be accompanied by an assessment of the arterial perfusion to the foot

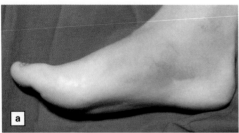

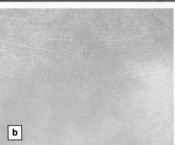

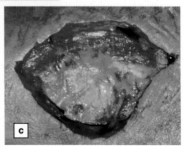

Fig. 5.13
(a) Cellulitic foot with patch of purple discolouration. (b) Close-up view of purple discolouration. (c) Same foot after debridement showing extent of subcutaneous necrosis.

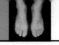

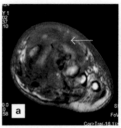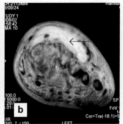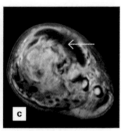

Fig. 5.14
(a) T1 sequence shows inflammatory mass (arrowed) but normal uptake in dorsum of foot. (b) High uptake in the dorsum on STIR sequence (arrowed). (c) Collection of fluid (arrowed) on the dorsum (post gadolinium). (With thanks to Dr David Elias and Dr Huw Walters.)

to evaluate the healing potential of surgical wounds. All of these patients will need urgent vascular investigation.

Perioperative care of neuropathic and neuroischaemic patients
On admission, these patients should be regarded as medical and surgical emergencies. The infected diabetic foot may require immediate surgical intervention

PREPARATION FOR SURGERY
The following investigations should be carried out:
- Full blood count and cross-matching
- Serum electrolytes and creatinine
- Blood glucose
- Liver function tests
- Electrocardiogram
- Chest X-ray.

Often it is difficult to assess how much debridement will be necessary and in some cases it may need to be accompanied by toe or ray amputation. Therefore, consent for these procedures should be obtained prior to operation.

An intravenous insulin sliding scale (Table 5.6) should be started. It is important to avoid veins in the lower limb as insertion of intravenous cannula into the veins of the foot can lead to ulceration,

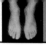

especially if the tip of the cannula goes into the subcutaneous tissues (Fig. 5.15).

The anaesthetist must be aware that virtually all of these patients will have autonomic as well as peripheral neuropathy, and respiratory reflexes may be diminished. Postoperative respiratory arrests have been reported. Careful anaesthetic attention, particularly in the recovery room, is necessary.

Insulin sliding scale

50 units soluble human insulin in 50 mL 0.9% sodium chloride

Blood glucose (mmol/L)	Infusion rate (units/h)
<4	0.5
4.1–9	1
9.1–15	2
15.1–19.9	4
>20	review and call doctor

Fluids

If blood glucose >11 mmol/L give sodium chloride 0.9%
If blood glucose ≤11 mmol/L give glucose 5%

Table 5.6
Insulin sliding scale. Adjust volume of fluids according to clinical state of patient.

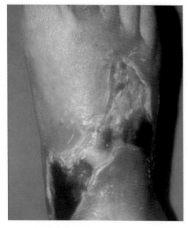

Fig. 5.15
Cellulitis and necrosis on dorsum of foot at infected intravenous cannula site.

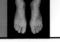

The anaesthetist should understand that debridement of the foot is not a rapid procedure such as incision and drainage for abscess, and therefore should anticipate at least 40 minutes operating time.

DURING SURGERY

- It is important that a meticulous wound exploration is carried out, with removal of infected sloughy tissue and laying open of all sinuses. It is rare to find a well-defined abscess
- The usual presentation is of heavily infected sloughy, grey tissue which needs to be removed down to healthy, bleeding tissue
- All dead tendon and necrotic tissue should be removed. Wide excision is necessary; small incisions with drains should be avoided
- Fragmented infected and non-bleeding bone should be removed
- Deep infected tissue should be sent urgently to the microbiology laboratory
- The wound should not be sutured but left to heal by secondary intention. A proflavine pack may be inserted into the wound.

In addition to debridement it may be necessary to perform a formal digital or ray amputation to establish drainage. The following techniques are used:

- Partial digital amputation may be performed for apical infection/osteomyelitis. Plantar and dorsal skin flaps are fashioned and the toe is disarticulated at the interphalangeal joint. If the toe is infected the wound is left open for delayed wound closure
- Hallux amputation may include removing the metatarsal head and a portion of the shaft in addition to the hallux (Faraboeuf procedure) to assist closure and render future ulceration less likely.
- Amputation of the lesser toes should be performed through the metatarso-phalangeal joint
- Ray amputation is performed for infection of a toe with limited spread to the forefoot and involves removal of toe and part or all of its corresponding metatarsal

- Open transmetatarsal, Lisfranc and Chopart's partial foot amputations are performed for extensive forefoot infections.

Further details of these operations are described in the companion volume to this book: A Practical Manual of Diabetic Foot Care (Blackwell Science, 2004).

AFTER SURGERY

- Continue the intravenous insulin pump postoperatively until infection is resolving. Then transfer to short-acting insulin three times daily with long-acting insulin at night
- Wound irrigation with a sodium hypochlorite solution (Milton) may be useful for the sloughy neuropathic foot. A 1 in 50 dilution of the neat 1% weight in volume solution of sodium hypochlorite is made by adding 20 mL of neat sodium hypochlorite to 980 mL of sterile water. Approximately 300–400 mL are irrigated through the wound, making sure to swab the edges of the wound and surrounding skin with normal saline at the end of the procedure. Milton irrigation should be stopped when the wound is no longer infected or sloughy (usually within five days)
- After surgery, the edges of the wound are debrided every three days and all callus, slough and non-viable tissue are removed. The wound is kept open and draining to heal from the base
- However, large surgical defects are now treated with VAC pump (see page 76) until they are granulating when they can either have split skin grafts applied or otherwise be left to heal by secondary intention
- When there is an initial fever preoperatively, the patient's temperature is a useful indication of his progress. A steady fall in temperature is expected over the subsequent three to four days. If this does not occur, then uncontrolled infection should be suspected. At operation, it is sometimes difficult to remove all infected tissue
- It is important to inspect the wound every day after the operation and if signs of infection recur then the patient may need further surgical intervention. Signs that the foot is settling include a decrease in erythema, less oedema, and a pink wound

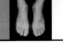

- Patients will need bedrest and it is wise to give prophylactic
  subcutaneous heparin. Low molecular weight heparin can be
  used except in patients in renal failure. Antithrombotic stockings
  should not be used on neuroischaemic feet. If used on a
  neuropathic foot, they should be folded back from the toe nails.

Vascular control

It is important to explore the possibility of revascularization in the
infected neuroischaemic foot. Improvement of perfusion will not only
help to control infection but will also promote healing of wounds if
operative debridement is necessary.

Urgent angiography should be carried out to detect the presence
of stenoses or occlusions. Duplex angiography or magnetic resonance
angiography (Figs. 5.16a and b) may initially be carried out.

Angiography

Most Stage 4 patients undergoing angiography will be in-patients.
Angiography is a safe procedure with few complications so long as a
rigorous checklist of patient details is carried out (see page 88).
Investigations should include:
- Full blood count, including a platelet count
- Blood coagulation indices
- Serum electrolytes and creatinine
- Blood grouping.

If the serum creatinine is above the normal range, then start
acetylcysteine therapy (see page 88). The patient should not be
dehydrated. Start an insulin sliding scale together with intravenous
fluids at least four hours before the procedure.

If the patient has previously been on warfarin then it may be
necessary to reverse its activity by administering vitamin K
parenterally. The patient should then be changed to an intravenous
unfractionated heparin infusion which is stopped two hours before
the procedure.

Post angiography, patients should be monitored closely, recording
blood pressure and pulse. There is a possibility of bleeding from the

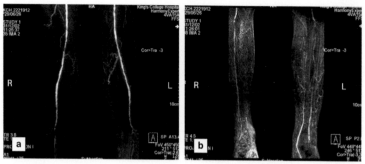

Fig. 5.16
Magnetic resonance angiography. (a) There is diffuse atheromatous disease of both superficial femoral arteries with an area of focal narrowing at the mid-level on the right. Both popliteal arteries are severely diseased. (b) On the right there is a single vessel, the anterior tibial, extending to the level of the plantar arch and it is severely diseased in the proximal aspect. There is reconstitution of posterior tibial at ankle level. On the left there is an occlusion of the tibioperoneal trunk with collaterals filling the more distal anterior and posterior tibial arteries.
(Courtesy of Dr Huw Walters.)

femoral artery injection site, which may not be immediately apparent. The pulse rate may not respond in the usual way to loss of intravascular volume because of autonomic neuropathy: therefore tachycardia may not be present. However, blood pressure will drop and an urgent blood count together with cross-matching for at least six pints of blood should be performed. Full resuscitation should immediately be carried out with haemodynamic monitoring. Most cases of bleeding resolve with blood replacement and tamponade themselves off spontaneously. A mass may become palpable in the lower abdomen but this may not appear until 5-6 hours after the procedure.

Continued hypotension despite adequate blood replacement is an indication for surgical exploration.

Angioplasty and arterial bypass
Angioplasty (Figs. 5.17a and b) is indicated in the treatment of single or multiple stenoses or short segment occlusions of less than 10 cm.

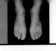

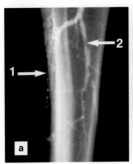 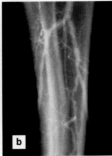

Fig. 5.17
Angioplasty (Courtesy of Dr H.Walters)
(a) Angiogram showing occlusion of anterior tibial artery (1) and stenosis of tibio-peroneal trunk (2).
(b) Post angioplasty. Anterior tibial flow has been restored and tibio-peroneal stenosis dilated.

If angioplasty is not possible because of long arterial occlusions, bypass should be considered.

If the infection is responding to conservative treatment, with resolution of cellulitis on intravenous antibiotics, then bypass, with its inherent risks, is probably not indicated. However, if operative debridement is necessary with amputation of a toe or ray, then arterial bypass may be necessary to achieve full wound healing.

Mechanical control

Patients with infected feet should not walk: they should be on bedrest and use crutches, Zimmer frame or wheelchair for trips to the bathroom.

Heels should be protected with a special pressure relieving mattress or regular and frequent turning in bed. After operative debridement in the neuropathic foot, off-loading of the postoperative wound may be achieved by casting techniques including Scotchcast boots and total contact casts. It may be necessary to cut a window in the cast (a 'windowed total contact cast') at the site of the wound in order to observe it closely.

In the neuroischaemic foot, non-weight bearing is advised until the wound is healed.

Metabolic control

It is important to make sure that there is no systemic, metabolic or nutritional disturbance to impair the response to infection and retard healing of wounds. Full blood count, serum electrolytes and serum creatinine and liver function tests should be checked. If serum albumin is <3.5 g/L, supplementary feeding with high energy drinks or via a thin bore nasogastric tube should be instituted under the supervision of a dietician.

In severe infections, considerable metabolic decompensation may occur. Full resuscitation is urgently required with intravenous fluids and intravenous insulin sliding scale which is often necessary to achieve good blood glucose control whilst the patient is infected. This is followed by a basal-bolus regimen of three times a day short-acting insulin before meals and long-acting insulin at night.

These are complex patients, and cardiac and renal function should be assessed. Echocardiography will identify patients with left ventricular dysfunction. This is expressed as the ejection fraction and a value less than 35% increases the risk of surgery. Close observation and monitoring of cardiovascular and renal function is essential to maintain correct electrolyte and fluid balance. Neuroischaemic patients should be regularly taking statins, angiotensin-converting enzyme (ACE) inhibitors and antiplatelet agents and these should be continued if the patient is admitted to hospital. Aspirin should not be stopped before angiography or angioplasty although if the patient is taking aspirin and clopidogrel, the latter should be stopped.

High blood glucose is associated with reduced white blood cell function, which improves when the blood glucose is lowered.

Controlling the great quartet of risk factors – hyperglycaemia, hypertension, hyperlipidaemia and smoking – is still important for Stage 4 patients.

Educational control

It is important for patients to know the warning signs of infection and to understand what to do once they have developed an infection.

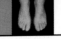

Patient information

WARNING SIGNS OF INFECTION

If a wound becomes

- Wetter than usual with increased amounts of discharge on the dressing
- Discoloured with redness, blueness or darker colour, or red streaks on the leg

you should be worried about infection.

Other signs of infection include

- Swelling around the ulcer
- If your foot becomes warmer than the other foot.

If you cannot see your foot clearly then someone will need to help you to check your foot for danger signs of infection.

The earlier an infection is treated the easier it is to control it. Always seek help the same day, as early as possible.

WHAT TO DO WHEN YOU HAVE AN INFECTION

- Your foot has developed an infection. This is a very serious problem which can destroy your foot
- Please stay in bed or on a sofa with your feet up
- If in bed, your heels need to be protected. Also, make sure your feet are not pressing against the end of the bed
- If you are allowed to sit out of bed on a chair, put your feet up on a stool covered by a pillow
- Contact the doctor or nurse at once if your leg becomes more painful or if you feel hot, shivery or unwell
- Some people with diabetes are particularly prone to develop infection. When you have recovered from this infection it will be necessary for you to keep a close eye on your feet in future, to prevent further episodes.

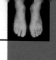

Chapter 6

Managing Stage 5: the necrotic foot

PRESENTATION AND DIAGNOSIS

This stage is characterized by the presence of necrosis (gangrene), which has grave implications, threatening the loss of the limb. It is important to limit the extent of necrosis and early diagnosis and intervention, even at this late stage, can save limbs. Necrosis can involve skin, subcutaneous and fascial layers. In the skin it is easily evident but in the subcutaneous and fascial layers it is not so apparent. Often the bluish-black discolouration of skin is the 'tip of an iceberg' of massive necrosis which occurs in subcutaneous and fascial planes, so-called necrotizing fasciitis (Figs. 6.1a and b).

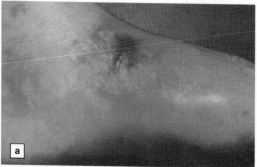

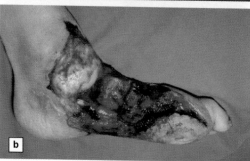

Fig. 6.1
(a) Cutaneous necrosis on medial surface of foot indicating severe underlying tissue destruction. (b) After debridement with extensive removal of necrotic tissue.

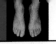

It is classified as either wet necrosis due to infection (Fig. 6.2) or dry necrosis due to ischaemia (Fig. 6.3). Purplish-black discolouration of the skin also occurs after bruising and is sometimes difficult to differentiate from early necrosis in the very ischaemic foot, although extensive bruising is usually associated with a history of trauma. Blood within a blister on a toe gives the toe a black appearance. Blue-black cyanosed toes and feet are seen in severe cardiac and respiratory failure. Shoe dye and the application of henna will result in black discolouration of the skin.

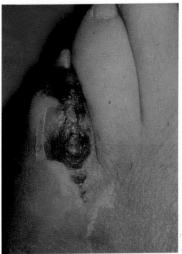

Fig. 6.2
Necrotic toe resulting from infection in neuropathic foot.

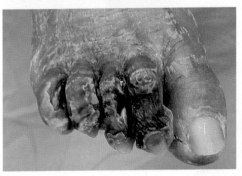

Fig. 6.3
Dry necrosis in Afro-Caribbean foot may be difficult to diagnose.

Wet necrosis

In wet necrosis, the tissues are grey, black, brown, white or greenish, moist and often malodorous (Fig. 6.4a). Adjoining tissues are infected and pus may discharge from the ulcerated demarcation line between necrosis and viable tissue.

Wet necrosis is secondary to a septic vasculitis (Fig. 6.4b), associated with severe soft-tissue infection and ulceration, and is the commonest cause of necrosis in the diabetic foot.

Dry necrosis

Dry necrosis is hard, blackened, mummified tissue and there is usually a clean demarcation line between necrosis and viable tissue (Fig. 6.3). It may be difficult to diagnose in the Afro-Caribbean foot.

Dry necrosis usually results from severe ischaemia secondary to poor tissue perfusion from atherosclerotic narrowing of the arteries of the leg, often complicated by thrombus and emboli. Necrosis is not usually due to a microangiopathic arteriolar occlusive disease, or so-called small-vessel disease.

Necrosis in the neuropathic and the neuroischaemic foot
Neuropathic foot

In the neuropathic foot, necrosis is almost invariably wet, and is caused by infection complicating a digital, metatarsal or heel ulcer,

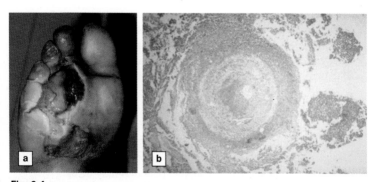

Fig. 6.4
(a) Wet necrosis of lesser toes and mid foot. (b) Septic vasculitis. Cross-section of digital artery showing lumen almost totally occluded by septic thrombus.

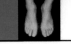

and leading to a septic vasculitis of the digital and small arteries of the foot. The walls of these arteries are infiltrated by polymorphs leading to occlusion of the lumen by septic thrombus (Fig. 6.4b).

Neuroischaemic foot
Both wet and dry necrosis can occur in the neuroischaemic foot.

Wet necrosis is caused by a septic vasculitis, secondary to soft-tissue infection and ulceration. However, in the neuroischaemic foot reduced arterial perfusion to the foot resulting from atherosclerotic occlusive disease of the leg arteries is an important predisposing factor.

Dry necrosis is secondary to a reduction in arterial perfusion and occurs in four circumstances:
- Severe chronic ischaemia
- Acute ischaemia
- Emboli to the toes
- End stage renal failure.

SEVERE CHRONIC ISCHAEMIA
Peripheral arterial disease usually progresses slowly in the diabetic patient, but eventually a severe reduction in arterial perfusion results in vascular compromise of the skin, often precipitated by minor trauma, leading to a blue toe which usually become necrotic unless the foot is revascularized.

ACUTE ISCHAEMIA
Blue discolouration leading to necrosis of the toes is also seen in acute ischaemia, which is usually caused either by thrombosis of an atherosclerotic stenosis in the superficial femoral or popliteal artery or emboli from proximal atherosclerotic plaques in the iliac, femoral or popliteal arteries.

It presents as a sudden onset of pain in the leg associated with pallor of the foot, quickly followed by mottling and slatey grey discolouration (Fig. 6.5). The diabetic patient may not get paraesthesiae because of an existing sensory neuropathy, which also reduces the severity of ischaemic pain and may delay presentation.

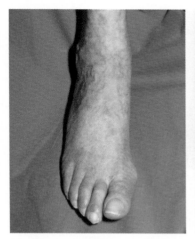

Fig. 6.5
Acute ischaemia–pale and mottled foot following sudden occlusion of superficial femoral artery.

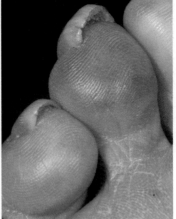

Fig. 6.6
Purple discolouration of fourth toe secondary to embolus.

EMBOLI TO THE TOES

Another cause of necrosis, particularly to the toe, are emboli (Fig. 6.6) to the digital circulation originating from atherosclerotic plaques in the aorta and leg arteries.

The initial sign may be bluish or purple discolouration which is quite well demarcated but which quickly proceeds to necrosis. If it escapes infection it will dry out and mummify. Microemboli present with painful petechial lesions in the foot that do not blanch on pressure.

END STAGE RENAL FAILURE

Digital necrosis is a relatively common problem in patients with advanced diabetic nephropathy and can occur in the absence of severe peripheral arterial disease and infection (Fig. 6.7). It may be precipitated by trauma.

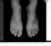

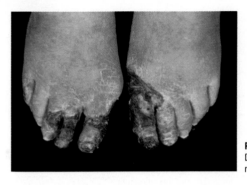

Fig. 6.7
Dry, well-demarcated necrosis.

MANAGEMENT

Patients should be admitted immediately for urgent investigations and multidisciplinary management. It is important to achieve:

- Wound control
- Microbiological control
- Vascular control
- Mechanical control
- Metabolic control
- Educational control.

Patients who present with necrosis, especially neuroischaemic patients, usually have severe multi-system disease and significant co-morbidities. They are often old and fragile and have cardiovascular disease and renal impairment. These diabetic patients can rapidly become very unwell leading to drowsiness and immobility. This renders them susceptible to pressure necrosis which can be disastrous.

If admitted to hospital, they are particularly susceptible to pressure necrosis of both heels and the sacrum. These areas should be examined often and pressure-relieving measures taken to prevent pressure necrosis. A pressure-relieving mattress should be used and if there is any degree of drowsiness the patient should be turned regularly. Heels should be protected in bed and this may need the application of a pressure relief ankle foot orthosis (PRAFO). Cardiac failure and renal impairment should be treated aggressively.

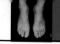

Wound control

Neuropathic foot

In the neuropathic foot, operative debridement is almost always indicated for wet necrosis. The main principle of treatment is surgical removal of the necrotic tissue, which may include toe or ray amputation or, rarely, transmetatarsal amputation. Although necrosis may not be associated with a definite collection of pus, the necrotic tissue still needs to be removed.

The diabetic foot does not tolerate the presence of infected necrotic tissue. In the neuropathic foot, this should be surgically excised as quickly as possible. Surgical procedures include extensive debridement and excision of necrotic soft-tissue and bone. In addition, a formal amputation may be necessary and this includes:

- Partial or total amputation of necrotic toes
- Ray amputation
- Transmetatarsal amputation
- Chopart or Lisfranc partial foot amputations
- Symes amputation.

Further details of these operations are described in the companion volume to this book: A Practical Manual of Diabetic Foot Care (Blackwell Science, 2004). In the neuropathic foot, there is good arterial circulation and the wound should heal as long as infection is controlled.

Very occasionally patients may not be suitable for or refuse operation, and the aim would then be to convert wet necrosis into dry by conservative treatment and intravenous antibiotics.

Neuroischaemic foot

In the neuroischaemic foot, wet necrosis should also be removed when it is associated with severe spreading sepsis. This should be done whether pus is present or not (Figs. 6.8a and b).

In cases when the limb is not immediately threatened, and the necrosis is limited to one or two toes, it may be possible to control infection with intravenous antibiotics and proceed to urgent revascularization and at the same operation perform digital or ray amputation.

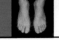

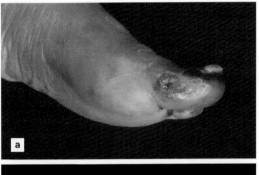

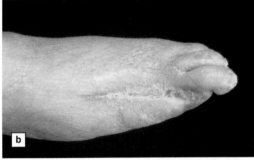

Fig. 6.8
(a) Necrosis of the toe with spreading cellulitis. (b) Foot healed after first toe amputation and distal bypass.

If angioplasty or bypass is not possible, then a decision must be made either to amputate the toes in the presence of ischaemia or allow the toes, if infection is controlled, to convert to dry necrosis and autoamputate. Surgical amputation should be undertaken if the circulation is not severely impaired, that is, a pressure index > 0.5 or a transcutaneous oxygen tension > 30 mmHg. The recent use of the VAC pump promptly applied to such post-operative wounds has encouraged healing in ischaemic limbs that cannot be revascularized.

Operative debridement

The preparation and principles of operative debridement are similar to that described in Stage 4. Patients will need full blood count, serum electrolytes and creatinine, blood grouping, chest X-ray and ECG. Consent should be obtained for the most extensive debridement anticipated, including digital or ray amputation.

It is important to remove all necrotic tissue, down to bleeding tissue, as well as opening up all sinuses. Deep necrotic tissue should be sent for culture immediately. Wounds should not be sutured. A foot with a large gaping wound following extensive tissue removal may be lightly held together by winding long strips of paraffin gauze around the foot; however, the strips should be cut through to accommodate swelling and must not prevent drainage of exudate. In the neuropathic foot, irrigation with 2% Milton (1 in 50 dilution – see page 117) may be useful for five days. Large wounds are treated with a VAC pump to encourage granulation. The VAC dressing should not be placed adjacent to an arterial anastomosis site for fear of disturbing the anastomosis and causing an arterial bleed. Skin grafting may be the best way to achieve healing of large tissue deficits (Figs. 6.9a and b). Ischaemic wounds are extremely slow to heal even after revascularization, and wound care needs to continue on an outpatient basis in the diabetic foot clinic, but with patience, outcomes may be surprisingly good.

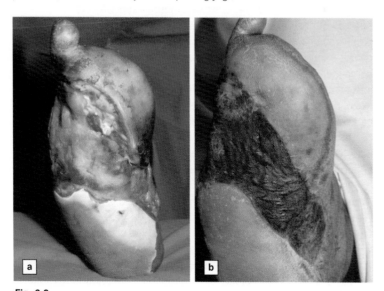

Fig. 6.9
(a) Large plantar defect. (b) A skin graft (pigmented skin) has achieved healing of a large plantar defect.

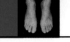

Free tissue transfer

Debridement of necrotic lesions of the foot often leads to severe tissue deficits. Management of these soft-tissue deficits is complex and skin grafts, local flaps and free tissue transfer have been used. In free tissue transfer, donor tissue from above the waist is utilised, particularly the muscle flaps, rectus abdominis and latissimus dorsi. The arteriovenous pedicle accompanies the transferred tissue and is anastomosed, usually to a pedal or tibial vessel, which is either a bypass graft or a native revascularized artery. These serve as the inflow tract for the free flap and anastomosis is achieved using microsurgical techniques. Free tissue transfer for limb salvage is a major undertaking in diabetic patients and should be carried out with caution in diabetic patients who may be of advanced age and have significant co-morbidities.

Autoamputation

Careful sharp debridement is performed along the demarcation line between necrosis and viable tissue to debulk dead tissue, drain pockets of pus and prevent accumulation of debris. Dry sterile dressings are used to separate necrotic toes from their fellows, for if necrosis is in direct contact with viable tissue, it can absorb perspiration and become wet. This provides an ideal culture medium for bacteria, and infection and necrosis can spread. Patients should not bathe to ensure that necrotic tissues are kept dry, since moistening necrosis may encourage infection.

Such neuroischaemic feet with dry necrosis may remain at Stage 5 for many months and are followed up until the necrotic toe drops off to reveal a healed stump (Figs. 6.10a and b).

Microbiological control
Wet necrosis

The microbiological principles of managing wet necrosis are similar to that of the management of infection in Stage 4. When the patient initially presents, send off deep wound swabs and tissue specimens for microbiology. Deep tissue taken at operative debridement must also go for culture.

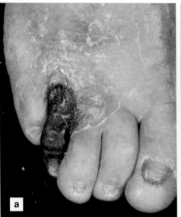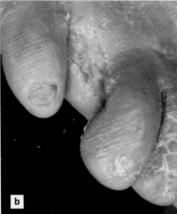

Fig. 6.10
(a) Dry digital gangrene in a neuroischaemic foot managed conservatively.
(b) Toe has autoamputated after 5 months.

Intravenous antibiotic therapy (amoxicillin 500 mg t.d.s., flucloxacillin 500 mg q.d.s., metronidazole 500 mg t.d.s. and ceftazidime 1 g t.d.s.) should be given. However, if the patient is allergic to penicillin, then clarithromycin 500 mg b.d. or vancomycin 1 g b.d. (dosage adjusted according to serum levels) may be used instead of amoxicillin and flucloxacillin. Antibiotic therapy should be adjusted when the results of cultures are available. Vancomycin will be needed for MRSA infections (Fig. 6.11).

Intravenous antibiotics can be replaced with oral therapy after operative debridement and when infection is controlled. On discharge from hospital, oral antibiotics are continued and reviewed regularly in the foot clinic. When the wound is granulating well and swabs are negative then the antibiotics are stopped.

Dry necrosis

When dry necrosis develops secondary to severe ischaemia, antibiotics should be prescribed if discharge develops or the wound swab is positive, and continued until there is no evidence of clinical or microbiological infection.

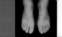

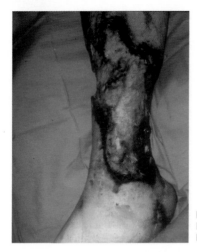

Fig. 6.11
Extensive necrotic wound following
MRSA infection.

When toes have gone from wet to dry necrosis and are allowed to autoamputate, antibiotics should only be stopped if the necrosis is dry and mummified, the foot is entirely pain-free, and there is no discharge exuding from the demarcation line.

Daily inspection is essential. Regular swabs should be sent for culture and antibiotics should be restarted if the demarcation line becomes moist or swabs grow organisms.

Vascular control

All neuroischaemic feet that present with necrosis must have Doppler studies to confirm ischaemia followed by Duplex arteriography to show stenoses or occlusions of the arteries of the leg. In wet necrosis, revascularization is necessary to heal the tissue deficit after operative debridement. In dry necrosis which occurs in the background of severe arterial disease, revascularization is necessary to maintain the viability of the limb.

When dry necrosis is secondary to emboli, a possible source should be investigated, and therefore the following should be performed:

- Electrocardiogram (ECG) to detect atrial fibrillation or recent myocardial infarct
- Ultrasound of abdomen to detect aortic aneurysm
- Arteriography of the lower limbs to detect atherosclerotic plaque in iliac or femoral arteries.

In some patients, increased perfusion following angioplasty may be useful. However, unless there is a very significant localized stenosis in iliac or femoral arteries, angioplasty rarely restores pulsatile blood flow to the foot which is necessary to keep the limb viable in severe ischaemia or restore considerable tissue deficits secondary to necrosis. This is best achieved by arterial bypass.

Patients will have cardiovascular disease and need preoperative assessment to maximise cardiorespiratory status. Peripheral arterial disease is common in the tibial arteries, and distal bypass with autologous vein has become an established method of revascularization (Fig. 6.12), in which a conduit is fashioned from either the femoral or popliteal artery down to a tibial artery in the lower leg, or the dorsalis pedis artery on the dorsum of the foot.

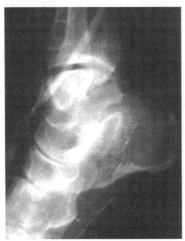

Fig. 6.12
Vein bypass seen passing across ankle to the dorsalis pedis artery.
(Courtesy of Mr. S. Fraser)

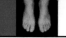

Patency rates and limb salvage rates after revascularization do not differ between diabetic patients and non-diabetic patients, and a more aggressive approach to such revascularization procedures should be promoted.

Postoperatively, the leg has wounds both where the graft has been inserted and from where the vein has been harvested (Figs. 6.13a and b). Wounds overlying the arterial graft must be kept free from infection otherwise the graft will block. Such wounds need regular cleaning and covering with dry sterile dressings, and any associated necrotic tissue which becomes bulky or moist should be gently debrided. Postoperative oedema is common and elevation of the leg is important. The patient should enter a graft surveillance programme.

Mechanical control

During the peri- and postoperative period, bedrest is essential with elevation of the limb to relieve oedema, but heels must be protected (Fig. 6.14).

After operative debridement of the neuroischaemic foot, especially when revascularization has not been possible, non-weight

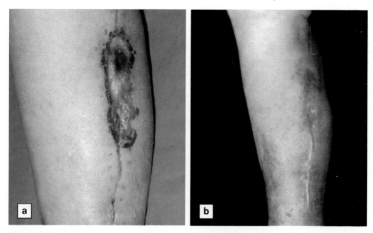

Fig. 6.13
(a) Distal bypass leg wound with slough and necrosis. (b) Leg shown in *(a)* healed after 1 year.

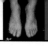

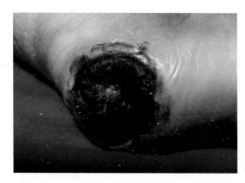

Fig. 6.14
Failure to protect heel from
pressure led to full-
thickness necrosis.

bearing is advised until the wound is healed. In the neuropathic foot,
non-weight bearing is advisable initially and then off-loading of the
healing postoperative wound may be achieved by casting techniques.

If necrosis is to be treated conservatively, by autoamputation,
which can take several months, then the patient needs a wide-fitting
shoe to accommodate the foot and dressings. Patients should walk
as little as possible. The Scotchcast boot (see Chapter 4) is very
useful for ischaemic patients with necrotic toes awaiting
autoamputation.

Metabolic control

When patients present with necrosis, in the background of severe
infection or ischaemia, they may be very ill, and will need close
metabolic and haemodynamic monitoring. Considerable metabolic
decompensation may occur, and full resuscitation is required with
intravenous fluids and intravenous insulin sliding scale which is often
necessary to achieve good blood glucose control whilst the patient is
infected or the leg severely ischaemic.

Patients will often have cardiac and renal impairment which will
need careful monitoring to optimize the regulation of fluid balance, so
as to avoid hypotension from underperfusion and hypertension and
peripheral oedema from overperfusion. Oedema is a potent cause of
impaired wound healing. Many patients have autonomic neuropathy
which may contribute to impaired blood pressure control and cardiac
arrhythmias.

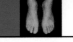

Nutritional impairment is denoted by a serum albumin of <3.5g/L. A high calorie diet should be instituted. A minimum of 1,800 calories per day should be ingested to avoid the negative nitrogen balance that could accompany the depletion of protein stores. Dietary advice should be obtained and nasogastric feeding nay be required. In patients with concomitant severe cerebrovascular disease and impaired swallowing, percutaneous endoscopic gastrostomy (PEG) feeding may be necessary.

Educational control

Patient information
Patients who develop necrosis need careful education including reassurance that much can be done to help them. We believe that practical and straightforward explanations are best. And advice should be given for when the patient is in hospital and at home.

IN HOSPITAL
- Your foot has developed a very serious problem
- Please stay in bed to keep your feet up
- Your heels need to be protected
- Move your feet about in the bed and try not to lie in the same position for long periods
- Make sure your feet are not pressing against the end of the bed

- If you are allowed to sit out of bed on a chair, put your feet up on a stool covered by a pillow.

AT HOME (FOR PATIENTS UNDERGOING AUTOAMPUTATION)

- Rest your foot, keep it up, and walk as little as possible
- You may want to obtain a wheelchair so that you can go out even before your foot has healed
- Your foot should be kept dry and covered with a dressing and bandage
- If you want to have a bath or shower you should cover your foot with a special wound protecting plastic bag to keep it clean and dry
- It is important to take great care of the condition of the skin. The skin of your feet (not immediately next to the black areas) should be kept clean
- Moisturising cream should be applied to prevent cracks. Neglected skin is a common cause of foot problems
- A nurse should visit regularly to clean, dress and inspect your foot and check your other foot as well for cracks, splits, dry skin or new ulcers
- Ask for help with household chores. You should be resting, not working
- Return to the foot clinic immediately (the same day!) if your foot becomes swollen, painful, develops an unpleasant smell or part of your foot changes colour or discharges pus.

Chapter 7

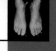

Managing Stage 6: the unsalvageable foot

PRESENTATION

Rehabilitation of the diabetic amputee is extremely difficult and is characterized by long stays in hospital. Only 25% of diabetic amputees will ever walk again. Morbidity and mortality associated with major amputation are very high. Major amputation therefore must not be taken lightly. It does not guarantee a future ulcer-free existence. However, it is sometimes inevitable in neuroischaemic patients. Major amputation may be necessary in the following circumstances:

- When pain is agonizing and cannot be controlled despite optimal analgesia, and no vascular intervention is possible
- When overwhelming infection has destroyed the foot
- When extensive necrosis, after a massive acute reduction in arterial perfusion, has inexorably spread up the foot (Fig. 7.1)

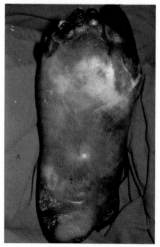

Fig. 7.1
Overwhelming necrosis secondary to popliteal artery thrombosis. The patient presented late because neuropathy reduced the pain.

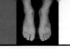

- In cases of unstable, inoperable Charcot ankle joint where attempts at external fixation have failed and internal fixation is not possible.

Major amputation in a neuropathic foot should be a very rare event and is usually necessary only when infection has irretrievably destroyed the foot. This should be preventable in most cases. A non-healing ulcer should not necessarily be an indication for major amputation.

MAJOR AMPUTATION
Preoperative care
Physical assessment of the patient is important. Cardiorespiratory status and metabolic control should be optimized. Patients should be encouraged to stop smoking. Malnutrition increases the risk of delayed wound healing. Weight loss and diminished appetite are common and patients should be seen by the dietitian.

The level of amputation should be carefully considered to ensure that there is sufficient perfusion to achieve wound healing, and, when possible, a below-knee amputation should be carried out as this will conserve the knee joint and aid the fitting of a prosthesis. Antibiotic prophylaxis should be used. Once major amputation is planned a lumbar epidural block with bupivicaine can be started 48 hours beforehand to relieve postoperative pain.

Perioperative care
A major amputation puts the remaining foot at great risk. The heel should be protected on the operating table.

Postoperative care
Patients who undergo an amputation often suffer from shock, disbelief and sadness. Patient and family need attention, support, sympathy and reassurance. Amputation wounds are often slow to heal in neuroischaemic patients. Infection should be treated aggressively but if there is poor arterial perfusion to the below-knee wound it may be necessary to convert it into an above-knee amputation.

Rehabilitation

Before the definitive prosthesis is issued, some patients may be suitable for mobility aids. The amputee mobility aid (AMA) is suitable for below and through-knee amputees only. The stump is supported and stabilised by an inflatable bag, which also assists in reducing oedema. The pneumatic postamputation mobility aid (PPAM aid) has an inflatable socket and is suitable for above-knee, through-knee and below-knee amputees.

The definitive prosthesis contains a stump sheath worn inside a customized thermoplastic socket fitted onto a modular prosthesis. Donning and doffing may be difficult for patients with neuropathic hands and poor eyesight.

Stump oedema may be a problem. Compression stump shrinkers provide good oedema control, both short and long-term.

Once healed, the stump should be inspected daily for skin breakdown, which should be cleaned, dressed and off-loaded until complete healing is achieved. Neuropathic stumps are prone to ulceration. This is preceded by callus which should be debrided with a scalpel. After amputation, the value of the remaining limb should not be underestimated: even if the patient never walks again he will need his leg to transfer from chair to bed and lavatory and thus maintain a little independence.

A major amputation will put the remaining foot at great risk of ulceration. The heel of the surviving foot should be protected on the operating table and postoperatively. Amputees undergoing rehabilitation should be provided with suitable footwear. The key for success is careful follow-up. Regular foot checks and preventive foot care are essential. There should be close links between the diabetic foot team, the rehabilitation team and ward staff. Everyone must understand the need to avoid trauma to the remaining foot at all costs. Major amputees are among the most high-risk of all diabetic foot patients.

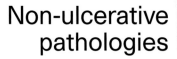

Chapter 8

Non-ulcerative pathologies

THE CHARCOT FOOT
Presentation

The term Charcot foot refers to bone and joint destruction that occurs in the neuropathic foot or rarely just the toe. It can be divided into three phases:

- acute onset
- bony destruction/deformity
- radiological consolidation and stabilization.

Acute onset

There is unilateral erythema and oedema and the foot is at least 2°C hotter than the contralateral foot (Fig. 8.1). There may be a history of minor trauma. The Charcot foot may follow injudicious mobilization after surgery or casting.

About 30% of patients complain of pain or discomfort. Rarely, pain may be very severe. X-ray at this time may be normal. However, a technetium methylene diphosphonate bone scan (Fig. 8.2) will detect early evidence of bony destruction. Early diagnosis is essential.

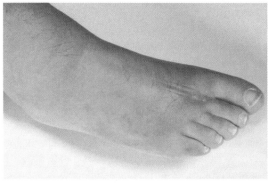

Fig. 8.1
The Charcot foot – acute stage. Redness and swelling.

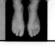

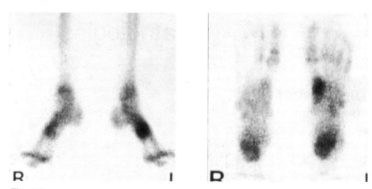

Fig. 8.2
Technetium diphosphonate bone scan showing increased uptake at the base of the first metatarsal of the left foot, indicating early bony damage despite normal X-ray.

Patients awaiting bone scan should be treated as if the diagnosis has been confirmed. Although patients with an early injury may appear to be developing a Charcot foot, it is not yet possible to differentiate between those who will resolve and not go on to develop a Charcot foot and those who will develop extensive bony destruction. For this reason, all patients with a history of trauma and redness, warmth and oedema should be offered treatment. If the problem is not a Charcot foot but a simple sprain, it will resolve rapidly. Magnetic resonance imaging is increasingly used to detect early intra-articular fractures not visible on X-ray.

It is important to differentiate between the red, hot, swollen Charcot foot and the red, hot, swollen cellulitic foot. Cellulitis is more likely in the presence of an ulcer which may show typical signs of infection (see Chapter 5). The swelling of the Charcot foot responds more rapidly to elevation than does that of the infected foot. If there is any doubt as to the correct diagnosis, antibiotics should be prescribed since the two conditions can sometimes be concurrent and this should be followed up by regular observation and further investigation of the foot. Gout and deep vein thrombosis may also masquerade as a Charcot foot.

The foot is protected within a total contact cast to prevent deformity. The patient may mobilize for brief periods. However, the patient is given crutches and encouraged to keep his walking to a minimum for at least four weeks. An alternative is the Aircast removable walker, but a cradled moulded insole should protect the sole. Such treatment if given early should help to prevent the second phase, that of bony destruction. Bisphosphonates may be helpful in the treatment of the Charcot foot but should be given early.

Bony destruction

Clinical signs are swelling, warmth, a temperature 2°C greater than the contralateral foot and deformities including the rocker-bottom deformity and the medial convexity. Ulceration can develop at these deformities and become infected and need surgical debridement (Figs. 8.3a and b). X-ray reveals fragmentation, fracture, new bone formation, subluxation and dislocation (Fig. 8.4a and b). These changes often develop very rapidly, within a few weeks of the onset.

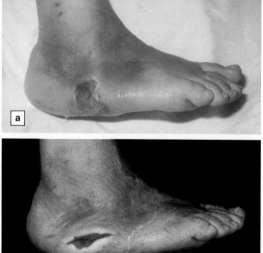

Fig. 8.3
(a) Infected ulcer with cellulitis in a Charcot foot. (b) Ulcer has been surgically drained.

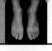

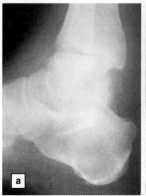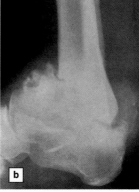

Fig. 8.4
(a) and (b) The Charcot foot; rapid destruction of ankle and subtalar joints within 8 weeks.

The aim of treatment is immobilization until there is no longer evidence on X-ray of continuing bone destruction and the foot temperature is within 2°C of the contralateral foot which can be measured with a skin thermometer. Deformity in a Charcot foot can predispose to ulceration, which may become infected and lead to osteomyelitis. This may be difficult to distinguish from neuropathic bone and joint changes, as on X-ray, bone scan or magnetic resonance imaging, appearances are similar. However, if the ulcer can be probed to bone, osteomyelitis is the more likely diagnosis.

Stabilization

The foot is no longer warm and red. There may still be oedema but the difference in skin temperature between the feet is less than 2°C. The X-ray shows fracture healing, sclerosis and bone remodelling. The patient can now progress from a total contact cast to a removable orthotic walker, fitted with cradled moulded insoles if necessary to accommodate a rocker-bottom or medial convexity deformity.

However, too rapid mobilization can be disastrous, resulting in further bone destruction. Extremely careful rehabilitation should be the rule, beginning with just a few short steps in the new footwear.

The patient rests for the remainder of the day and monitors the foot. If there is no increase in warmth, swelling and redness then he can walk a few more steps the next day and very carefully build up to a reasonable amount of walking. Finally, the patient may progress to bespoke footwear with moulded insoles.

The rocker-bottom Charcot foot with plantar bony prominence is a site of very high pressure. Regular reduction of callus can prevent ulceration. If the deformity is severe, a surgical procedure such as ostectomy of plantar prominences may help.

The most serious complication of a Charcot foot is instability of the hind foot. This can lead to a flail ankle on which it is impossible to walk without fixation. This condition can sometimes be managed with a Charcot Restraint Orthotic Walker (CROW) which is a bespoke bivalved outer shell to support the foot and ankle (Figs. 8.5a and b). Many patients progress to an ankle foot orthosis and custom made boots in the long term.

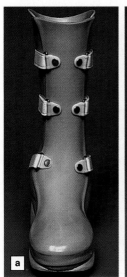
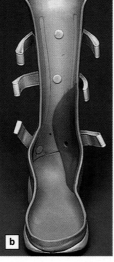

Fig. 8.5
(a) Anterior view of the CROW (with front piece). (b) Anterior view of the CROW with removal of the front piece to show interior. Extra internal padding (blue) has been added to cushion the vulnerable malleolar areas.

Alternatively, reconstructive surgery and arthrodesis of the hind foot, with a long-term ankle foot orthosis, has resulted in high levels of limb salvage (Fig. 8.6). The favoured method for arthrodesis is open reduction with internal fixation. Recent advances in limb salvage surgery, especially when infection of the joint fusion site is suspected, have included the use of external stabilization with an Ilizarov frame coupled with internal operative stabilization.

Surgery should never be undertaken lightly. Potential complications include:

- Infection
- Non-union
- Progressive bone and joint destruction
- Recurrent deformity.

The timing of surgery is important. Intervention should be delayed until the acute bone destructive phase has settled down. Very careful rehabilitation and careful fitting with optimal footwear and orthoses is essential. Details of the operations for Charcot osteoarthropathy are given in the companion volume to this book: A Practical Manual of Diabetic Foot Care (Blackwell Science, 2004).

Occasionally the knee joint will develop Charcot osteoarthropathy and patients will present with swelling of the knee. Patients with a Charcot knee will almost certainly have had a previous history of Charcot foot.

PATHOLOGICAL (NEUROPATHIC) FRACTURE

The usual presentation is of a red, swollen foot with relatively little pain. There may be a history of trauma. The fracture may be the initial bony change in the development of a Charcot foot (Figs. 8.7a and b). Commonest sites of fracture include metatarsal head, shaft or base.

Initial X-ray may be normal, but in the presence of excessive swelling, a technetium methylene diphosphonate bone scan is advisable. Fractures do not heal at the same rate as in non-diabetic patients. Fractures in the diabetic patient should be treated with plaster cast, supported by crutches and/or wheelchair. Duration of casting should be greater for diabetic patients compared with non-diabetic patients. Healing should be confirmed by X-ray, and skin

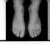

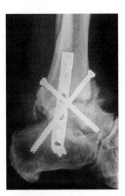

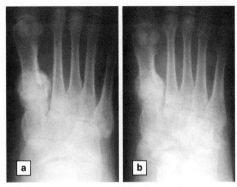

Fig. 8.6
X-ray of reconstructed Charcot hind foot and ankle (Courtesy of Dr. M Myerson).

Fig. 8.7
(a) Fractured base of first metatarsal. (b) The development of a Charcot foot with disorganization of the tarsus and fragmented navicular and cuboid.

temperature at site of fracture should be within 2°C of the similar site on the contralateral foot. Healing of metatarsal fractures may take up to six months, and in some cases full union is not attained.

PAINFUL NEUROPATHY
Presentation
This is a singularly disagreeable complication of diabetes. The patient develops severe burning pain, worse at night, paraesthesiae and contact discomfort, sometimes rendering him unable to wear normal clothing. Symptoms may also include interrupted sleep, restless legs, cramps, depression and weight loss. It may be precipitated by optimizing diabetic control, or by periods of poor control.

Management
General approach
Reassure the patient that intense pain improves within two years. Sympathetic support is essential and patients need regular appointments to monitor their pain and try new strategies if previous attempts at relieving pain are ineffective. It is essential to optimize diabetic control. Insulin may be needed.

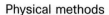

Physical methods

Very simple techniques, such as wearing silk pyjamas or nylon tights under clothes, may relieve contact discomfort. A bed cradle holding the bedclothes off the legs may be helpful. Application of cold water may be soothing: some patients even keep a bucket of cold water by the bed in case they wake in pain.

Applying OpSite film to painful areas may reduce pain and contact discomfort. Transcutaneous electrical nerve stimulation (TENS) machines can be used to block the pain.

CAPSAICIN

This topical cream releases substance P, a peptide neurotransmitter involved in pain transmission at various levels. Acute release often causes transient burning or stinging with erythema followed by insensitivity to painful thermal or mechanical stimuli which lasts several hours. Capsaicin is applied sparingly in a thin layer, three or preferably four times a day. It may cause temporary stinging and burning but these effects usually disappear within 2–6 weeks. The treatment should be persisted with because the analgesic effect can take up to six weeks to develop. There are no significant side-effects.

Drugs

In the first instance, simple analgesics (aspirin, paracetamol and mild opiates, singly or in combination) should be tried. For disturbed sleep, hypnotics may be prescribed. If necessary, stronger analgesics may be given, such as dihydrocodeine or tramadol.

ANTICONVULSANT DRUGS

Gabapentin is a useful therapy. The dosage can be rapidly increased over seven days to reach 1800mg as the maximum dose. This drug has very few side effects: occasionally it causes somnolence and dizziness. However, it is generally well tolerated and has no significant interactions with other drugs. The dosage should be reduced in renal failure. Recently, pregabalin has been introduced. It has a similar action to gabapentin with a similar side-effect profile. The dosage can be increased over two weeks from 75 mg b.d. to 300 mg b.d. Carbamazepine, valproate and phenytoin may be useful. Carbamazepine can be started at 100 mg once or twice daily and increased up to the maximum tolerated dosage (usually 800–1000 mg/day). Sodium valproate (100–500 mg 1–3 times daily) and phenytoin (100–400 mg 1–2 times daily) may be helpful.

TRICYCLIC ANTIDEPRESSANTS

Imipramine or amitriptyline may relieve burning pain. Commence with a low dose, gradually increased according to symptomatic response. Imipramine is slightly less effective than amitriptyline but has fewer side-effects. With imipramine, begin at 25–50 mg at night and increase by 25 mg increments on alternate days. The drug should be taken at night both for its relief of pain and for its sedative effect. The addition of a phenothiazine, such as fluphenazine, enhances the analgesia but may make possible hypotension worse.

In the USA duloxetine hydrochloride (Cymbalta) has received FDA appproval for treatment of painful neuropathy.

OPIOIDS

Opioids may be used for short periods especially at night when patients have severe pain and find it difficult to sleep.

ANTIARRHYTHMIC DRUGS

These are rarely used. Lidocaine is given by intermittent intravenous infusion and may provide relief for several days. Mexiletine often has unacceptable side-effects although dosages of 450 mg a day significantly reduce burning pain and paraesthesiae without causing cardiovascular side-effects.

Epilogue

Our many years of experience in managing the most high-risk diabetic feet at King's lead us to conclude that neuropathic feet are demanding yet forgiving. The excellent blood supply means that the neuropathic foot has a great capacity for healing, when properly managed. Neuropathic feet only come to amputation as a result of untreated, rapidly ascending infection. The neuroischaemic foot is far more likely to come to major amputation. In some cases, despite great efforts on the part of the multidisciplinary team, the foot inexorably develops necrosis and comes to a major amputation. However, health care practitioners should not regard poor outcomes as inevitable: in many cases, amputation can be prevented or delayed for several years, even in severely ischaemic diabetic feet. However, the leeway for error is greatly diminished: the neuroischaemic foot is not a 'forgiving' foot.

It is the authors' strong belief that the natural and optimal forum for managing the high risk diabetic foot, be it neuropathic or be it neuroischaemic, is the multidisciplinary diabetic foot clinic, where access to investigations, admission to hospital beds, urgent surgery, and advice and support from other members of the team are available without delay. It is also the optimum forum in which to provide useful follow up and continuity of care. The diabetic foot remains one of the most difficult challenges of 21st century medicine and needs lifelong surveillance. All healthcare professionals should be persuaded to refer diabetic foot patients early. The diabetic foot patient deserves to be managed by a multidisciplinary team within a diabetic foot clinic and it is the role of the diabetic foot clinic team, through good times and bad times.

"To strive, to seek, to find, and not to yield."
Alfred, Lord Tennyson: *"In Memorium"*

Appendix

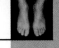

Problems of differential diagnosis

Further Reading

A Practical Manual of Diabetic Foot Care. Edmonds M, Foster AVM, Sanders L. Blackwell Science, Oxford, 2004.

Levin & O'Neal's The Diabetic Foot. Bowker JH, Pfeifer MA, (Eds), 6th Edition. Mosby Year Book, St. Louis, 2001.

The Foot in Diabetes. Boulton AJM, Connor H and Cavanagh PR, eds, 3rd Edition. John Wiley & Sons, Chichester, UK, 2000.

International Consensus on the Diabetic Foot. The International Working Group on the Diabetic Foot, 1999 and 2003.

The Diabetic Foot. Medical and Surgical Management. Veves A, Giurini JM, Logerfo FW (Eds). Humana Press, New Jersey, 2002.

Prevention and management of foot problems: Clinical Guidelines for Type 2 Diabetes. National Institute of Clinical Excellence, 2004

Index

Page numbers in **bold** represent tables, those in *italics* represent figures.

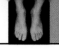